Vitamin C:
Its Molecular Biology
and Medical Potential

To my Ann

Vitamin C:
Its Molecular Biology
and Medical Potential

Sherry Lewin

Department of Postgraduate Molecular Biology,
North-East London Polytechnic,
London, England

1976

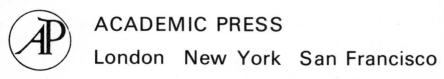

ACADEMIC PRESS

London   New York   San Francisco

A Subsidiary of Harcourt Brace Jovanovich, Publishers

ACADEMIC PRESS INC. (LONDON) LTD.
24/28 Oval Road,
London NW1

United States Edition published by
ACADEMIC PRESS INC.
111 Fifth Avenue
New York, New York 10003

Library of Congress Catalog Card Number: 76 016979
ISBN: 0 12 446 3509

Printed in Great Britain by
William Clowes & Sons Limited
London, Colchester and Beccles

Preface

Considerable evidence has been presented in the last forty years that "high" intake of ascorbic acid—nutritionally termed vitamin C—results in beneficial effects in many individuals; yet several contrary conclusions have been reported. The conditions reported as beneficially affected range widely and include the common cold, cardiovascular defects, high levels of cholesterol, some diabetic conditions, several viral diseases, and states of mental depression and schizophrenia. Naturally two questions arise: why is it that so many investigators and ex-sufferers consider that these benefits are real, while others feel that these reports cannot be substantiated; and how are the outstandingly versatile activity and medical potential of high intake of ascorbic acid (as reported) to be explained at the molecular level? This monograph covers the background and provides answers to these questions.

It is generally considered that although a certain intake of ascorbic acid is essential for health, humans are unable to biosynthesize it, and this deficiency has received considerable attention. Two aspects in particular have been debated, namely why ascorbic acid is not biosynthesized by humans, and what is the daily dose required.

On the basis of *in vitro* examination of tissue homogenate extracts (but not allowing for possible mitochondrial contributions), Burns (1957) concluded that man, monkey and guinea pig are unable to convert L-gulonolactone to L-ascorbic acid, and that this is the missing step in the biosynthesis in the livers of these species which makes them dependent on exogenous L-ascorbic acid for their vitamin C requirements. Chatterjee *et al.* (1961) concluded that there exists an *additional* missing step, namely that performed in other species by the enzyme glucuronolactonase in converting D-glucuronolactone to L-gulonolactone. More specifically Burns (1956), Stone (1966) and Chatterjee *et al.* (1975) considered that the "missing step" is due to gene deletion.

Two points must be highlighted at the very outset. *First*, it has not been proved beyond reasonable doubt that it is L-gulonolactone oxidase which is the "missing step". To note but one indication,

Baker *et al.* (1962) found that several individuals could metabolize both D-glucuronolactone and L-gulonolactone to ascorbic acid. Any defective—not necessarily missing—step is therefore likely to be sited earlier on in the biosynthetic sequence of ascorbic acid, probably in the enzyme aldonolactonase, which is required for the conversion of the acid form into the lactone. Considerations will be presented which assist in resolving this issue. *Second*, weighty experimental and theoretical considerations will be advanced in favour of the thesis that vitamin C deficiency in a number of species including humans is not due to *total* inability to biosynthesize ascorbate, but rather to a very limited biosynthetic ability which normally cannot be stepped up to meet the minimum metabolic/physiological requirements.

The size of the required daily dose has, for quite some time, been subject to considerable controversy. The recommended doses by various governmental medical boards have been of the order of 30 mg to 125 mg. In contrast, the Szent-Gyorgyi/Stone/Pauling school (e.g. Pauling, 1970; Stone, 1972) has advocated the view that humans require daily multi-gram quantities of ascorbic acid for full expression of their maximum potential for health and for ability to resist present-day stresses and bodily malfunctions, and they have advanced powerful considerations in support of this thesis. However, the rationale behind the thesis of the need for, and beneficial effect of, large intake of ascorbic acid relies on empirical observations, calculations of the intake of the vitamin by other animals requiring it, and on the ability to produce higher quantities of the vitamin in other animals—such as rats—as a response to increased stress conditions. The *rationale* for specific benefits following high intake of the vitamin has not been expressed in terms of biochemical/molecular biological mechanisms. Neither have the considerable variations in benefits been explained.

Considerable literature exists covering the need for the lower ascorbic daily dose. This will therefore not be considered here unless relevant to the overall pattern I have developed in this book where I collate new work—some of which is my own unpublished work—with many experimental biochemical/physiological/clinical observations dispersed throughout the literature, which so far have not been collated within a single framework. This monograph evaluates the uses and any limitations of the multi-gram daily dose of the vitamin.

The pattern of observations and the rationale for them presented in this book cover direct, intermediate and indirect activities of ascorbate. The first of these deals with beneficial effects resulting directly from the physicochemical properties of the ascorbic system—including those of the ascorbic free radical (AFR) and the ability of ascorbate to react directly with histamine thereby introducing anti-histamine activity and offsetting biochemical stress. Intermediate effects include those affecting enzyme systems, and the indirect effects include those which arise from contribution of the ascorbic system to the inhibition of cyclic AMP-phosphodiesterase (PDE) and upkeep of higher concentrations of cyclic AMP and cyclic GMP. Evaluations of the effect of intake of the vitamin have in the past suffered from some lack of appreciation of the difference between the quantity ingested and that absorbed as well as from pitfalls present in the methods of assay of ascorbate present in the tissues. Attention has been drawn to pitfalls such as rapid deactivation of the vitamin under specific conditions and in particular to my recent findings that the ascorbate ring is hydrolytically ruptured by cyclic AMP phosphodiesterase. In this connection I suggest an additional procedure which enables differentation between the vitamin and its delactonized product.

The original cause of the researches leading to the writing of this book arose from an incident involving an unclear request to my wife. I had been in the habit of taking a daily dose of 50 mg of synthetic vitamic C for many years. This did not prevent the onset of angina and eventual coronary, in 1967, as a result of being subjected to considerable stress in my work. After leaving hospital, I was subject to anginal symptoms on bending to open and shut the garage gates. One day, being rather preoccupied, I asked my wife to "buy me some vitamin C tablets". My wife bought the vitamin C, but the tablets were the 1 gm effervescent variety, as they were the only vitamin C tablets visible on the counter at the chemists. At the time this seemed rather an excessive dose; but rather than waste the tablets, I took one early each morning. I then noted a temporary absence of anginal symptoms following the exertion accompanying the opening of the garage gates. I checked the phenomenon; it was somehow related to the timing of the intake of the vitamin C tablet. I then followed the regime of taking the tablets about an hour before each exertion and found myself increasingly free from subsequent anginal unease. Later I noted that the incidence, severity and duration of the heavy colds and blocked nose and sinusitis to which I had been subject previously were effectively reduced by the intake of two to three daily doses—each of c. one gm of ascorbic acid. Further, the outbreak of cold-sores (herpes) to which I was subject two to three times a year no longer occurred. Naturally, I became deeply interested in the *modus operandi* at the molecular level of the prophylactic and therapeutic effects of mega-intake of the vitamin. Consequently I undertook an extensive investigation into the theoretical and practical aspects of the problems involved, as a result of which this monograph emerged.

I must stress that this book is not a text-book which sets out to incorporate and evaluate scattered information in the field of ascorbic acid utilization. To do so would require an encyclopedia of many thousands of pages since the available literature on fields in which ascorbic acid participates involves over ten thousand publications. In this monograph I have concentrated on marshalling published data and unpublished work of my own within patterns explaining the effect of intake of vitamin C in what have often been termed mega-doses, i.e. well above the recognized daily allowance of 10 mg to 125 mg.

Many new ideas are presented here. In this connection it must be emphasized that for a new proposal to be considered permissible, it must be stereochemically and energetically admissible. I have therefore made appropriate use of molecular model building and energetic considerations in evaluating the admissibility of the new concepts. It must also be emphasized that the analysis and patterns presented in this monograph, although they explain many conditions in which mega-intake of ascorbic acid can be beneficial and also point to unexplored paths, have by no means exhausted all the ways and means by which the vitamin exercises its full potential. Much more research is required in order to evaluate the precise limits of beneficial effects and possible negative and even adverse effects in some individuals with particular genetic characteristics. Biochemical individuality can differ significantly; variations are bound to be encountered. It is therefore desirable, in fact essential, to evaluate individual needs and limitations.

It is my hope that the analysis presented here will aid greater appreciation of the various ways in which high intake of ascorbic acid can activate/deactivate different metabolic/physiological paths, and that it will thereby contribute to more precise formulations of future investigations in the field, particularly in respect of problems connected with vitamin C assay and biochemical individuality.

Since there are many aspects to vitamin C activity as well as numerous interrelationships between the many direct and indirect effects, it has proved difficult to deal with all associated points in the section on a particular use of ascorbate. Some restatements were inescapable. To decrease repetition considerable cross-referencing has been necessary.

A bibliography has been incorporated in the book, which gives the reader a brief outline of past developments and their medical effects, as well as listing sources of information which although relevant could not be dealt with in the content of the various chapters.

In the title of this book the term Molecular Biology was chosen—not Biochemistry, although fundamental biochemical aspects are effectively covered. Biochemistry and Molecular Biology are considered to overlap in many areas. The term Molecular Biology was chosen because of a differentiation which appears to me to be apposite. Biochemistry can be likened to the spinning of yarn in that it covers the field of manufacture of biological molecules and in particular macromolecules. The weaving of particular patterns from the spun yarns bears a resemblance to the further state of molecular biology in which biochemical molecules participate in weaving the biological pattern. Here the biological pattern, in the weaving of which ascorbate participates, is the ultimate in the significance of its activities.

I should like to thank M. Black, P. Marshall, G. Stubbs and R. Stoker for assisting me in checking and re-checking some experimental observations I have recorded in this monograph. I should also like to thank Dr. L. Ellis for drawing my attention to a number of publications, and Dr. H. Caplin for discussions. I must however stress that I bear sole responsibility for the new ideas and concepts presented in this book.

This book is dedicated to my wife, but for whose constant and unstinted help progress towards its completion would have been much slower.

October, 1975   S. LEWIN

Contents

Part I

Chemical and biochemical reactivity

Introduction

The potential of the ascorbic system when ingested in multigram daily dosage raises the problem of how it is possible for such a comparatively small molecule to participate in so many activities and to possess such an extensive range of prophylactic and therapeutic potentials. The reaction of many scientists and, in particular, that of some members of the medical profession, has been scepticism, and even incredulity, often accompanied by strong opposition to the use of this compound in pharmacological doses. It is therefore essential to examine in depth the physico-chemical characteristics of the ascorbic system and to evaluate its potential to affect enzymatic as well as hormonal activities, since these must increase extensively the range of action.

Before embarking on this exercise it is relevant to point to a parallel case in respect of range of influence, that is, that of the comparatively small molecule of 3',5'-cyclic AMP. Subsequent to its discovery by Sutherland (1956), cyclic AMP was found to possess such a widespread potential of activity in relation to hormonal and enzymatic paths that it was rightly termed a "second messenger". Indeed, cyclic AMP and cyclic GMP are now known to influence so many biological activities—including cellular multiplication and differentiation—that had they not been repeatedly proven to possess these potentials, scepticism in respect of their seemingly incredibly wide, yet now established, activities would have been scientifically reasonable. It is relevant, even at this early stage, to point out that ascorbic acid is capable of enhancing an increase in the concentration levels of both cyclic AMP and cyclic GMP and thus indirectly affecting an extensive range of physiological activities.

Let us consider first the basis for the thesis that the smaller doses of vitamin C—in the range of 50 mg to 100 mg total daily—medically recommended for avoidance of the symptoms of scurvy, do not meet the optimal requirements for prophylaxis and treatment of the biochemical stresses to which humans are exposed. Various consider-

1

ations have been put forward in favour of this thesis. The most logical arguments can be presented as follows:

First, it has been shown experimentally that individuals or animals who do not synthesize their own vitamin C and who are subject to biochemical stress or bodily malfunctions display depleted levels of vitamin C in particular tissues, such as leucocytes or adrenals (see for example, Goth and Littman, 1948; Waldo and Zipf, 1955, Hume *et al.*, 1972) compared to those individuals who are not subjected to such stress (for reviews see, for example, Goldsmith, 1961; Pauling, 1970; Stone, 1972). However, increased vitamin C levels in the tissues follow high intake of vitamin C (Kübler and Gehler, 1972) and such intake results in increase in resistance to malfunction (Spero, 1973; Yew, 1973; Coulehan *et al.*, 1974).

Second, animals capable of synthesizing their own vitamin C requirements have been shown to increase their synthesis multifold—and in some cases several hundred-fold—when exposed to bio-chemical stresses such as drug intake (e.g. Longenecker *et al.*, 1940; Conney *et al.*, 1961). Assuming that there is physiological co-oper-ation of animal activities, it is reasonable to argue that if animals which can meet their own vitamin requirements by synthesis switch over to *multifold* production, this is because they now require—on being subjected to biochemical stress—higher quantities of the vitamin. This argument is cogent provided it can also be shown that higher ascorbate concentrations in the tissues can offset the cause of the stress. Now, biochemical stress is known to be associated with over-production and secretion of histamine. It follows that if it can be shown that ascorbate can "neutralize" histamine ·i.e. act as an anti-histamine agent—it will have a biochemical anti-stress function. As will be shown subsequently (see section 1.3.4.2) ascorbate reacts with histamine under laboratory conditions; it has also been found to display anti-histamine effect clinically (see section 4.4.6).

It is apposite to highlight here one particular effect of mental stress, that is of increased adrenaline and noradrenaline biosynthesis. This increase enhances oxidative formation of the corresponding highly toxic adrenochrome and noradrenochrome. Ascorbate pro-tects both hormones from the oxidation and also reduces them, thereby tending to inhibit toxicity. The utilization of ascorbate increases correspondingly with increase in the stress conditions. Sufficiently high ascorbic acid intake should mitigate the effects of stress.

Third, the presence of comparatively high concentrations of vitamin C in tissues which are concerned with response to biochemical stress—such as adrenals, leucocytes and pancreas (for tabulated values see, for example, section 4.3)—is indicative of its requirement for both immediate use and storage in physiological defence mechanisms and normal hormonal paths.

Hence, man—who is not capable of meeting his minimal vitamin C requirements by synthesis—should, when exposed to biochemical stress and corresponding higher vitamin C requirements, ingest correspondingly multifold quantities of the vitamin so as to reduce the probability of incurring body malfunction.

Once the above arguments and conclusions are accepted, several questions arise of which the most prominent are:

First, how can a small molecule such as vitamin C potentiate so many physiological and defence mechanisms?

Second, what are the paths via which the vitamin can express its potential?

Third, what side effects, if any, exist?

Two different approaches can be followed in answering these questions. One would begin by collecting and classifying all the experimental evidence concerning the effect of intake of mega quantities, and then attempt to construct a pattern which would be stereochemically and energetically admissible in respect of the potential of the ascorbic system. A different approach would be to consider the potential of all the relevant physiochemical properties of the ascorbic system and then assess the impact they could make on the human system by exerting specific influence on its physio-logical activities. Now, extensive documentation of various physio-logical influences of the ascorbic system has been carried out. However, despite this, these influences have not been collated within an overall framework. For example, the participation of the ascorbic system in several enzymatic reactions, such as the hydroxylation of lysine and proline in the formation of collagen, and in the hydroxyl-ation of thymidine (for review see Barnes and Kodicek, 1972) and in the formation of noradrenaline from dopamine (e.g. Levin and Kaufman, 1961) has been traced through to the molecular level. However, these evaluations do not extend to the much wider range of ascorbate-enhanced physiological activities, which are beneficial in such apparently widely different fields as cardiovascular malfunction, insulin deficiency, the common cold, cancer, chemical toxicity, allergy and depressed mental states. The common denominator(s) have appeared elusive until recently.

Following extensive re-examination of the overall field, and using the second approach to the elucidation of the *modus operandi* of the ascorbic system, I have concluded that the beneficial effects of high intake of ascorbic acid can conveniently be evaluated if the resultant effects are considered in two main categories—namely activities which result from direct action, including those in which the ascorbic free radical is involved, and activities which result from secondary actions via paths primarily controlled by hormones. The latter category can be further divided as proceeding either via the raising of the concentration levels of cyclic nucleotides and hormonally involved paths *or* via effects on enzyme systems. It is this second category which enables the use of mega quantities of ascorbic acid to exercise influence over a much wider overall field than the direct activity, thereby extending the ability of the biological system to resist biochemical stresses—so common in modern society—on a very wide front.

Chapter 1

Structures and characteristic properties
of the ascorbic system

1.1. Structure

The chemical and structural characteristics of L-ascorbic acid* can be described as follows:

The molecule is an α-keto-lactone with a formula of $C_6H_6O_8$; molecular weight of 176.13 daltons containing a double-bond between the C-2 (or α) and the C-3 (or β) carbons, and an acid-ionizing group in water, at *c.* pK 4.19. These characteristics are accommodated by the structure given below.

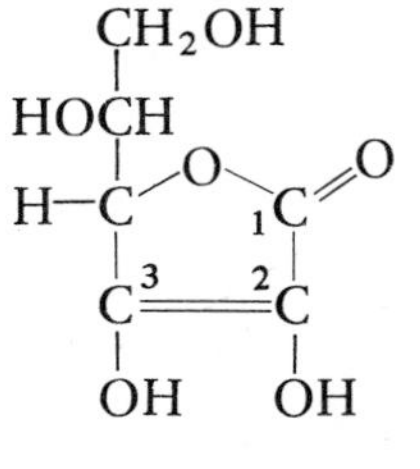

A photograph of a correctly-proportioned space-filling molecular model is given in Fig. 1.1.

The ring (lactone) representation was deduced as a result of physicochemical considerations; it has also been confirmed by magnetic measurements and molecular orbital considerations.†

The ring-structured ascorbic acid is formed from its open chain form by digestion with 8% HCl at 50°C (Haworth and Hirst, 1933). The ascorbate anion is formed on addition of alkali in equivalent

---

* D-ascorbic acid cannot replace L-ascorbic acid biologically.

† For references concerning structure and formulation see, for example, references (a) and (i) in Bibliography III.

5

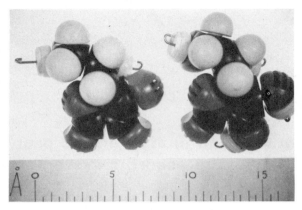

Fig. 1.1. Photograph of correctly proportioned space-filling molecular models (constructed from CPK atomic models) of the ascorbic acid and dehydroascorbic molecules displaying their hydrophobic areas (top areas with the white covalently bound hydrogens). Dehydroascorbic is on the left, and ascorbic acid is on the right.

quantities to an ascorbic acid solution. The alkali should be added slowly to avoid transient local rises in pH values to above $c.$ 9, as this would favour transient formation of the double negatively charged anion which decomposes comparatively quickly. The pH of Na ascorbate solution is $c.$ 7.6; the slight alkalinity is due to the weak acid nature of ascorbic acid (see section 1.2.3).

1.2. Physicochemical properties

Ascorbic acid and ascorbate possess a double-bond between C-2 and C-3 as well as existing in a ring configuration. The former parameter confers upon them the properties of optical absorbance and optical rotation. The latter contributes also to optical rotation.

1.2.1. Optical absorbance

The optical absorbance spectrum of the ascorbate anion differs clearly from that of ascorbic acid.

(a) *Ascorbate*. The optical absorbance spectrum of ascorbate has been determined in several laboratories. It is generally agreed that the ascorbate has a peak value at between 265 nm and 266 nm. The value determined in this laboratory is 265.5 nm ± 0.3. The value of ϵ_{max} as variously given in the literature ranges between 7500 and

16,650 (the latter value having been determined by Hewitt and Dickes, 1961). These values are rather low. Measurements carried out in this laboratory* have shown—under strict *anaerobic*† conditions—a continuing drop in absorbance in aqueous solutions at low ionic strengths of 10^{-4} to 10^{-3}. The drop can be attributed to (i) auto-oxidation catalysed by traces of multivalent cations, such as Cu

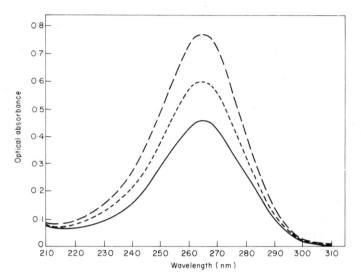

Fig. 1.2. Effect of time on the optical absorbance spectrum of sodium ascorbate under anaerobic conditions. Na ascorbate = 50 μM; pH 6.1; 25°C; 1 cm optical path length. (– – – – –) 9 minutes after preparation of the solution; ($\cdots\cdots$) 70 minutes after preparation of the solution; (———) 130 minutes after preparation of the solution. The solution was prepared from equivalent quantities of pure ascorbic acid and $NaHCO_3$, while bubbling N_2 free from O_2 and CO_2, using conductivity water.

and Fe, present in concentrations as low as 1 in 300,000 in the purified ascorbic acid samples used, and (ii) the effect of light present during preparation of the solutions.‡ The drop is illustrated in Figs. 1.2 and 1.3.

---

* Lewin, S. (1974a, and unpublished observations).

† Under *aerobic* conditions both rate and extent of oxidative deactivation of ascorbate are considerably enhanced (e.g. Morton, 1942).

‡ Search of the literature revealed other work where the exposure to light resulted in breakdown of ascorbate (e.g. Hendrickx and DeMoor (1962a, b)).

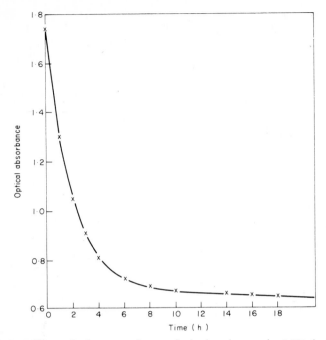

Fig. 1.3. Effect of time on the optical absorbance in 10% (w/v) sucrose solution in tap-water, pH 7.27 at 25°C under *aerobic* conditions. 0.6 mM ascorbic acid; 266 nm; 0.2 cm optical path length.

By using EDTA, or citrate or phosphate (as complexing or chelating agents), working in very dim light and strictly anaerobic conditions, significantly higher values were obtained. The value obtained using freshly prepared ascorbate solutions (pH values 7.4 to 7.6 at 10°C) in over 10^{-3} ionic strength in 0.01% EDTA was 20,400 ± 400 at 265 nm ± 0.3.

Increasing ionic strength under anaerobic conditions resulted in decreased rate of fall off in the value of absorbance. At 10^{-2} ionic strength and higher, the values were stable for several hours, at 10°C. Increased concentrations of glycerol or of other comparable non-electrolytes were found to stabilize the ascorbate.

Following these and other tests for stability of ascorbate solutions, it was found advisable to prepare fresh solutions, under N_2 free from O_2 and CO_2, in dim light. Freezing of stock solutions at low temperatures (e.g. −70°C) was helpful, but as the number of intermediate operations increased, increasing degree of instability was noted.

(b) *Ascorbic acid.* The highest ϵ_{max} values reported for ascorbic acid in acidified solutions (HCl or metaphosphoric, pH *c.* 1.5) were at λ_{max} 244 nm. Hewitt and Dickes (1961) give 10,500, while Lawendel (1956, 1957) gives the value of *c.* 11,900 to 12,220 in presence of sorbitol.

(c) *Dehydroascorbic (DHA).* DHA is transparent in the region of 230 nm to 280 nm, but has a weak absorption ϵ_{max} = 720 at 300 nm (Mattock, 1965).

1.2.2. Optical rotation

The optical rotation of ascorbate was determined by Herbert *et al.* (1933) as $[\alpha]_{5780}^{18°}$ = +116° in neutral aqueous solution, and in acid solution (N/20 HCl) as $[\alpha]_{D}^{18°}$ = +22°. However, no rechecked data appear to have been published for various other temperatures for the optical rotatory dispersion spectrum of ascorbate or ascorbic acid.

The optical rotatory dispersion spectrum of ascorbate was determined in this laboratory* using spectropolarimetry;† the method was found more sensitive than that of optical absorbance. The optical rotation values have been used to compare the relative stabilities of ascorbate solutions under anaerobic conditions at different concentrations and ionic strengths and under aerobic conditions. Thus, the initial value for the optical rotation of 10^{-2} M Na ascorbate solution, at 37°C and 365 nm, under anaerobic conditions was determined as +0.0376°; this value dropped to +0.0357° after 21 hours, i.e. a proportional drop of (0.0019/0.0376) = 0.0505. Using a 10^{-3} M ascorbate solution, under the same experimental conditions, the initial value of +0.038° dropped to +0.012 after 21 hours, i.e. a proportional drop of (0.026/0.038) = 0.68; this is a much greater drop in optical rotation than that displayed by the 10^{-2} M Na ascorbate solution.

This comparison is typical of the numerous results obtained in this laboratory showing that decreased ascorbate concentration (or decreased ionic strength) results in increased instability of the ascorbate solution under anaerobic conditions.

Aerobic conditions result in more pronounced changes in the values of the optical rotation, in line with oxidative processes taking place. For example, using a 10^{-3} M ascorbate solution, under the same

---

* All solutions were prepared in distilled and deionized water under anaerobic conditions (using N_2 free from O_2 and CO_2) unless otherwise stated.

† Lewin, S., Marshall, P. and Stubbs, G., unpublished observations.

experimental conditions as before, the initial reading was +0.023°.*
This fell to +0.003° in 21 hours, i.e. a proportional drop of
(0.020/0.023) = 0.87.

1.2.3. Ionization

Ascorbic acid ionizes in two stages as the pH of its aqueous
solution is raised on addition of alkali. At 37°C the first pK value is
4.18, and the second pK value is 11.6 (Karrer *et al.*, 1933; Borsook
et al., 1937). Kunler and Daniels (1935) give the respective values as
4.12 and 11.51. Birch and Harris (1933) determined the respective
values at 16 to 18°C as 4.17 and 11.57. The ionizations take place at
the C-2 OH and the C-3 OH sites.

1.2.4. Oxidation-reduction and its potential

1.2.4.1. *Oxidation to the dehydroascorbic entity*

Oxidation can be attained by the use of several agents, e.g.
2:6-dichlorophenolindophenol,   N-bromosuccinimide,   bromine,
iodine and mercuric chloride. The oxidation-reduction path of
ascorbate to dehydroascorbic is shown in part of Fig. 1.4. The
existence of an intermediate oxidation compound with semiquinone
properties—between ascorbate and DHA—has been established by
several investigators using electron spin resonance (ESR) measurements and other methods (e.g. Piette *et al.*, 1961; Yamazaki *et al.*,
1960; Yamazaki and Piette, 1961; Lagercrantz, 1964). This compound has been given several names, e.g. monodehydroascorbate
(MDHA) or semidehydroascorbate (SDA). Because of the free radical
nature of the compound it will be referred to in this book as the
Ascorbic Free Radical (AFR). See also sections 1.3.5 and 2.2.3.

1.2.4.2. *Redox potential*

A mixture of ascorbic/dehydroascorbic constituents exhibits a
redox potential. The value of +0.058 v and the variation of the redox
potential value with pH were determined by Ball (1937) over the
temperature range of 25 to 30°C. At pH 7.4—the value approxi-
mating to the blood of normal individuals—the potential is somewhat

---

* The lower reading—compared with the previous anaerobic values of +0.038—may be
attributed to aerobic oxidation of the solution during its preparation and while awaiting
instrument standardization.

lower, approximately by 10 mv. The standard redox potential of AFR/L-ascorbate—E'_0(pH 7.0)—was determined as +0.34 by Everling *et al.* (1969); the value of +0.32 was obtained by Weis (1975).

1.2.5. Stability and the effect of ionic strength and of bulk-water activity

1.2.5.1. *Stability of the ascorbate anion*

The optical absorbance peak region is due to the double bond between C-2 and C-3. Hence, reduction in optical absorbance value can be ascribed to corresponding loss of the double bond. The hypochromic changes and the ORD changes taking place in neutral solutions of ascorbate under anaerobic conditions—described previously—are indicative of the instability of the ascorbate anion in solutions of low ionic strength.

Instability of *aerobic* ascorbate solutions when multivalent cations are present has generally been attributed to cation catalysis of oxidation of the ascorbate anion. On these lines, the ability of EDTA to counter the changes has been explained as due to cation-chelating activity. However, in the *absence of oxygen*, no aerobic oxidation of ascorbate should be possible. This suggests that other deactivating factors, such as simultaneous anaerobic oxidation-reduction of two ascorbate molecules when catalysed by a multivalent ion (possibly similar to the Cannizarro reaction) may contribute. Several mechanisms are possible. One possible mechanism utilizing Fe^{++}/Fe^{+++} may be*:

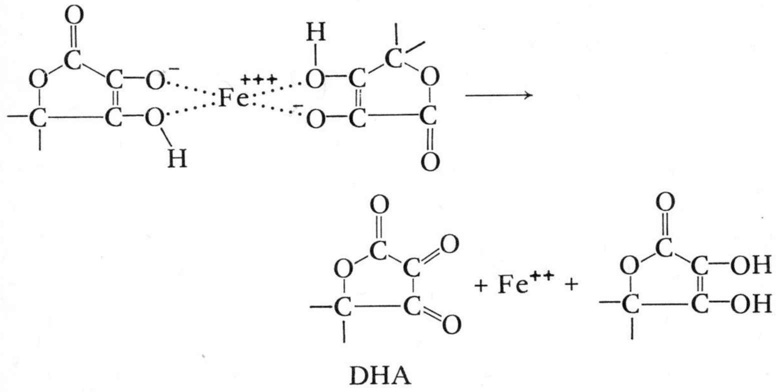

$$+ Fe^{++} + \qquad (1.1)$$

DHA

---

* See, however, Géro and LeGallic (1952), for involvement of Cu^{++}; see also Barr and King (1956) for γ-ray induced anaerobic and aerobic oxidations of ascorbic acid in presence of Fe^{++}.

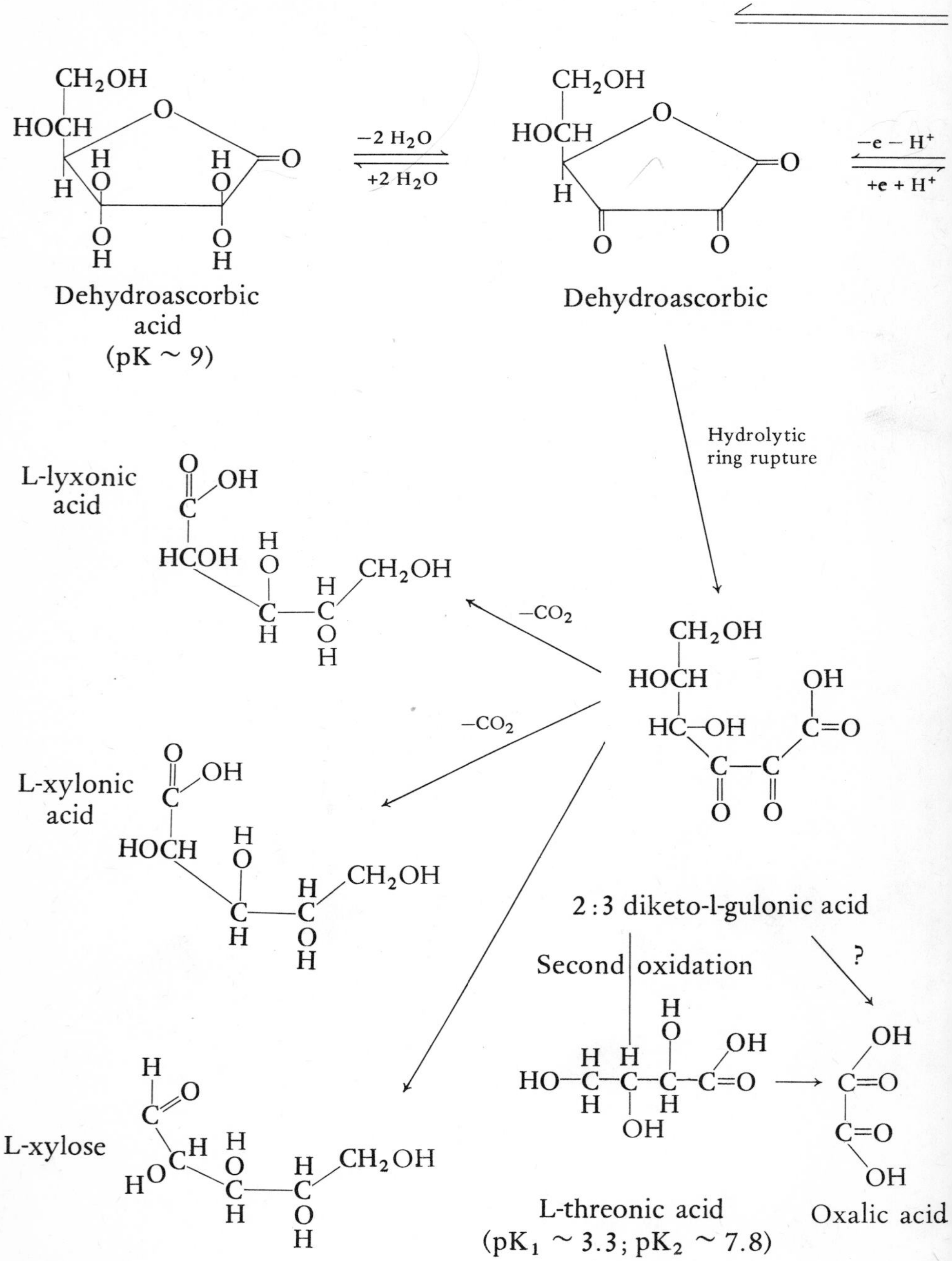

Dehydroascorbic
acid
(pK ~ 9)

$-2 H_2O$
$+2 H_2O$

Dehydroascorbic

$-e - H^+$
$+e + H^+$

Hydrolytic
ring rupture

L-lyxonic
acid

$-CO_2$

L-xylonic
acid

$-CO_2$

2:3 diketo-l-gulonic acid

Second oxidation

L-xylose

L-threonic acid
(pK$_1$ ~ 3.3; pK$_2$ ~ 7.8)

Oxalic acid

First oxidation (1 Ox. atom or I_2)

Reduction by W_2S

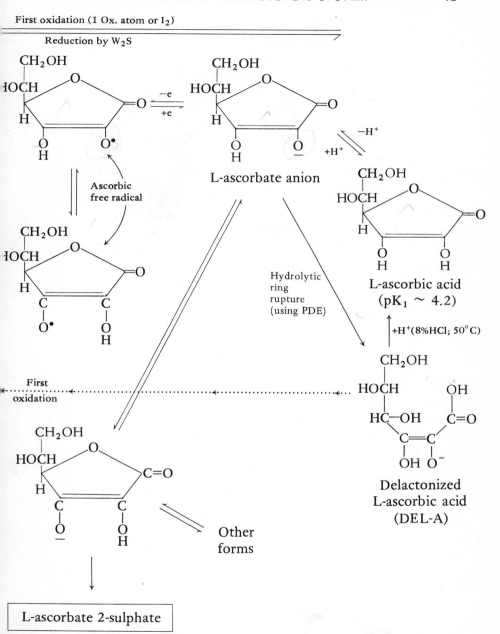

Fig. 1.4. Ascorbic acid and its products.

The loss of the double-bond on formation of DHA can—at least in part—explain the drop in optical absorbance; the repeated findings that under anaerobic conditions the drop does not necessarily reach zero absorbance value can be explained in terms of a limited oxidation-reduction and also as being associated with hydrolytic rupture of the lactone ring, where the open chain form possesses a lower absorbance. The increased stability with increasing ionic strength could at first sight be attributed either to reduction in the electrostatic field strength or to an association of non-ascorbate anions with multivalent cations present. It is worthwhile considering the two alternatives:

Reduction in electrostatic field strength: On ionization, the γ-lactone ring of the vitamin is subjected to considerable electrostatic stress—which is barely present in the acid form—between the newly established negative charge on the (C-2) O^- group and the negative end of the dipole of the carbonyl group, thus

$$
\begin{array}{c}
\quad\ |\quad O \quad \overset{\delta^+}{} \ \overset{\delta^-}{} \\
-\!\overset{|}{\underset{|}{C}}\diagup \ \diagdown \overset{}{\underset{|}{C}}\!=\!O \\
C\!=\!C \\
\quad\ \overset{|}{O}\quad\ \overset{|}{O}{}^- \\
\quad\ H
\end{array}
$$

An association with *multivalent* cations would tend to reduce this repulsion, but this would involve the ascorbate entity in oxidation-reduction changes resulting in decreased optical absorbance. The electrostatic repulsion could also be reduced by increasing ionic strength which intrinsically weakens all electrostatic repulsions, thus enhancing ascorbate stability.

Elimination of the catalytic activity of multivalent cations by association with non-ascorbate anions or by complex formation. The ability of multivalent cations present to associate with ascorbate can be offset by overriding association with non-ascorbate ions (such as Cl^- originating from the higher concentrations of NaCl introduced to give higher ionic strengths), thus

$$Fe^{+++} + 6Cl^- \rightleftharpoons [Fe^{+++}6Cl^-]^{---} \tag{1.2}$$

My findings that ascorbate in concentrations of over $5 \times 10^{-2} M$ displays increasing stability cannot be explained in these terms. This indicates that alternative (i) is more likely to *express* the stabilizing effect of increasing ionic strength on ascorbate solutions. The above indication should not however be given over-weighting, since another possibility exists, namely that deactivation at low ionic strength arises from water attack, as outlined below.

1.2.5.2. *Effect of activity of bulk water*

There are two ways in which the reaction of water with ascorbate may be formulated. Both depend on the freedom of the individual water molecules to undergo reaction. Bulk-water consists of a

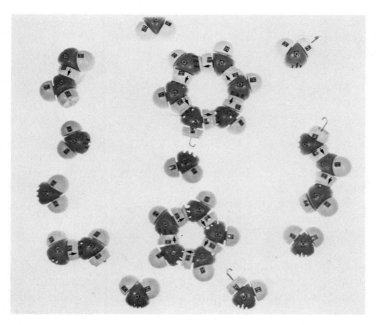

Fig. 1.5. A photograph of correctly proportioned space-filling molecular models (constructed from CPK atomic models) representing associations of water molecules in equilibrium with "free" water molecules.

mixture of numerous equilibria which comprise three-dimensional and two-dimensional structures which may be schematically depicted as in Fig. 1.5.

In very dilute solutions the activity of water is pronounced but with increasing ionic strength or with concentrations of neutral substances which can combine with or increase the extent of water-structuring, the number of free water molecules is correspondingly decreased. At low ionic strengths—and low concentrations of

water-combining or water-structuring entities—the probability increases that water will interact with ascorbate in the following two
ways, thus

Elimination of the double-bond

$$\begin{array}{c} \diagdown \\ \mathrm{C}\!=\!\mathrm{C} \\ | \quad | \\ \underline{\mathrm{OH}} \ \ \mathrm{O} \end{array} \ + \ \mathrm{H_2O} \quad \longrightarrow \quad \begin{array}{c} \mathrm{H} \\ \mathrm{H} \ \ \mathrm{O} \\ | \quad | \\ \mathrm{C}\!-\!\mathrm{C} \\ | \quad | \\ \underline{\mathrm{OH}} \ \ \mathrm{O} \end{array} \qquad (1.3)$$

Hydrolytic rupture of the lactone-ring structure

$$\begin{array}{c} | \quad \mathrm{O} \quad \diagup\! \mathrm{O} \\ \mathrm{H}\!-\!\mathrm{C} \quad \diagdown\! \mathrm{C} \\ | \qquad | \\ \mathrm{C}\!=\!\mathrm{C} \\ | \qquad | \\ \mathrm{O} \quad\ \ \mathrm{O} \\ \mathrm{H} \qquad \underline{\ } \end{array} \ + \ \mathrm{H_2O} \quad \longrightarrow \quad \begin{array}{c} \quad \mathrm{OH} \quad\ \ \mathrm{OH} \\ | \diagup \qquad | \\ \mathrm{H}\!-\!\mathrm{C} \qquad \mathrm{C}\!=\!\mathrm{O} \\ | \qquad\quad \diagup \\ \mathrm{C}\!=\!\mathrm{C} \\ | \qquad | \\ \mathrm{O} \qquad \mathrm{O} \\ \mathrm{H} \qquad \underline{\ } \end{array} \qquad (1.4)$$

The observations of Lawendel (1956) that both sorbitol and
mannitol in *high concentrations* exert a marked stabilizing effect on
ascorbic acid in aqueous solution are in accord with the thesis of
water involvement, since these substances associate effectively with
water thereby reducing the concentration/activity of individual water
molecules.

The activity of multivalent cations, such as Fe^{++}/Fe^{+++} (and the
suppression of their effect by addition of chelating agents such as
EDTA) can be integrated within an overall scheme in which the
water molecules associated with the cation display a free radical
activity (as H_2O^+) thereby assisting formation of the ascorbic free
radical (AFR) followed by formation of the dehydroascorbic entity;
see section 1.3.5.7.

1.2.5.3. *Overview of the stability of ascorbate and its detection*

In reviewing the stability of the ascorbate ion, it is apposite to
disentangle the following intrinsic contributions to instability:

Stereochemical strain owing to polar repulsive forces: These are
conducive to hydrolytic rupture of the ring.

Activity due to the double-bond: This is conducive to auto-
elimination by (i) oxidation, and (ii) water attachment to the

double-bond; see section 1.2.5.2. The auto-destructive forces are enhanced by the presence of multivalent cations, and by exposure to light and oxygen.

The symptoms of deactivation include reduction in the values of the optical parameters and increase in acidity (as a result of acidic products being formed on further oxidation, e.g. threonic and oxalic acids), or a reduction in acidity as a result of the formation of DHA (which has a higher pK value than ascorbic acid), or of hydration of the double bond (which reduces the pK value of the original OH group).

1.2.5.4. *Stability of the dehydroascorbic entity*

The dehydroascorbic entity resulting from the oxidation of ascorbate was found to have a pK value of *c.* 9 (Herbert *et al.*, 1933). This ionization can take place only as a result of hydration of the anhydrous form (see Fig. 1.5), since the latter does not possess an ionizable OH group either at C-2 or C-3. Borsook *et al.* (1937) concluded that DHA is highly unstable in aqueous solution, and that its "half-life" *in vitro* at the temperature and pH of the tissues lasts only a few minutes.

1.2.6. Lowering of the interfacial tension

Planar structures favour two-dimensional water associations at the expense of three-dimensional water associations thereby causing a lowering of the interfacial tension (Lewin, 1974a). Ascorbate possesses an essentially planar-ring-structure assisted by the siting of the carbonyl group and the double bond orientation in the same plane, as can be appreciated from Fig. 1.1; in addition it possesses a hydrophobic section. These two factors contribute to its ability to lower the interfacial tension. Indeed, 10^{-3} to 10^{-2} M ascorbate solutions lower the interfacial tension of water/air by *c.* 10 to 15 dynes per cm, depending on the temperature and composition of the solution. The effect was noted experimentally by Künzel (1941), and was computed on theoretical grounds (Lewin, 1974a) and confirmed experimentally. For example, a 10^{-2} M sodium ascorbate aqueous solution at $37°C$ attains the value of 55 ± 3 dynes per cm under anaerobic conditions.

The potential to lower the interfacial tension in biological activities is considered in section 2.4.

1.2.7. Complexing ability of the ascorbate anion

The ascorbate anion possesses the ability to form a complex with metallic cations,* as distinct from its complementary electrostatic association with cations. One way in which this activity can be diagrammatically represented is:

$$(1.5)$$

Several metallic ions, e.g. Fe^{+++} and Cu^{++} possess the capacity for

---

* The approximate values of the formation constants of 1:1 complexes of ascorbate with Ca and Sr in barbital buffer at pH values 7.2–7.3 and 25°C are respectively 0.19 and 0.35. Cf. the corresponding values for citrate as 3.16 and 2.85 (Schubert and Lindenbaum, 1952).

forming complexes with ascorbate. The effect can readily be demonstrated by the displacement of the titration curves of ascorbate in pH regions around the pK value, where the hydrated metallic ions do not undergo hydrolytic ionization.

1.2.8. H... bonding capacity

1.2.8.1. *Types of H... bonding*

The monovalent ascorbate anion possesses both an H... donor group (OH)—also capable of H... acceptance—and a $-C-O^-$ H... acceptor group, thereby enabling the molecule to participate not only in H... bonding in general, but specifically in simultaneous H... donation and H... acceptance. In contrast the anhydrous form of dehydroascorbic has no H... donor groups in its ring. However, the *hydrated* form of the dehydroascorbic can, by virtue of its OH groups on the C-2 and C-3 sites, be presumed to possess activity in both H... donation and H... acceptance.

These characteristics, the resonance potential entailed in the double bond between the C-2 and C-3 sites, and the negative end of the dipole of the carbonyl group, endow this section of the ascorbate with an enhanced potential for both unidirectional and complementary-two-dimensional double H... bonding activities, as follows:

1.2.8.2. *Unidirectional double H... bonding*

This can be illustrated by an interaction between the guanidinium group of arginine and the corresponding section of the ascorbate ring. The two N—H groups of the guanidinium act as H... donors, while either the ascorbate section

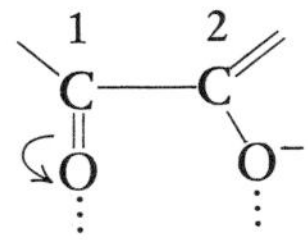

or the ascorbate section

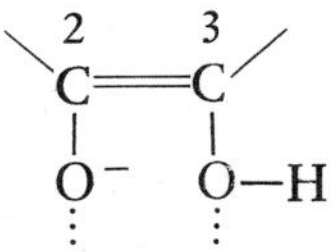

(a)

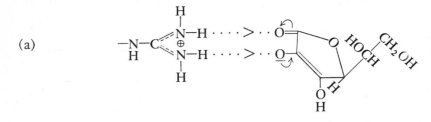

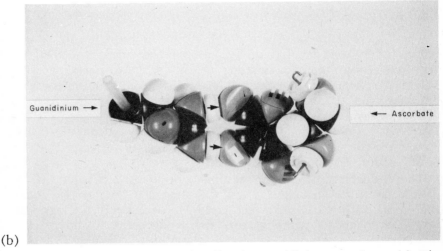

(b)

Fig. 1.6. Unidirectional H... bonding in guanidinium ascorbate. (a) Diagrammatic representation. (b) Correctly proportioned space-filling molecular representation.

acts as H... acceptor. The former is illustrated diagrammatically in Fig. 1.6a, and using correctly proportioned space-filling molecular models is represented in Fig. 1.6b. It is difficult to allocate relative probabilities of bonding to the respective associations in this scheme. On the one hand, the negative end of the dipole should be a more potent H... acceptor than the oxygen of the OH group. However, the resonance associated with the double bond could endow the oxygen of the OH group with an equal or a greater H... acceptance potential.

1.2.8.3. *Complementary H... bonding*

Using correctly proportioned space-filling molecular models, it can readily be shown that the C—O⁻ and the adjoining C—OH group can participate in complementary H... bonding with corresponding H... donor and H... acceptor groups suitably located in another molecular

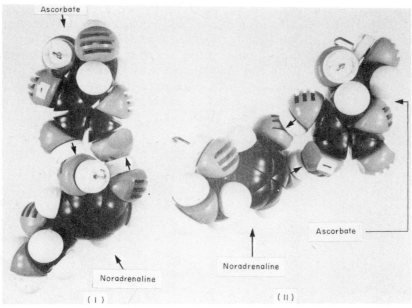

Fig. 1.7. (a) Schematic representation of two stereochemically and energetically complementary H... bondings between adrenaline and ascorbate. (b) Molecular model representation of stereochemically and energetically permissible complementary H... bonding between noradrenaline and ascorbate.

species. This can be used to postulate the formation of an association between the 3'OH and 4'OH groups of catecholamines—such as adrenaline and noradrenaline—and the relevant section of the ascorbate entity. Diagrammatically, this can be represented as in Fig. 1.7a, and using molecular-models as in Fig. 1.7b.

Such H... bonded associations should protect both constituents from oxidation. This expectation is in line with the findings of Leach *et al.* (1956) that ascorbate inhibits the oxidation of adrenaline in plasma, and with the commercial practice of utilizing ascorbic acid as a preservative for adrenaline (Hoffer and Osmond, 1963). For absorption spectra of adrenaline-ascorbate see Beauvillain and Sarradin (1948).

1.3. Chemical reactivity of the ascorbic/dehydroascorbic system

1.3.1. Interrelationships of ascorbic acid and its derivatives

The interrelationships of ascorbic acid and its oxidized derivatives are given in Fig. 1.4. Consider the reason for the greater stability of the double-bonded ring structure of the acid as compared to the open-chain form. It can be computed that the decrease of entropy associated with the former can be compensated by the decreased electrostatic repulsion (compared with open-chain forms where the negative ends of the dipoles would exert significant electrostatic repulsion) and by the increase in entropy of the water resulting from the formation of the lactone. Comparison of the three ring-structures diagrammatically represented below indicates that form I, which is the accepted structure of L-ascorbic acid, should possess the least electrostatic repulsion.

The formation of the ascorbate anion from the acid form is likely to involve ionization of the C-2 OH group because of the tendency to electron displacement towards the oxygen of the carbonyl group, thus $\rangle C=O$. However, the resultant repulsion between the negative end of the dipole of the carbonyl group and the (C-2)O⁻ area would favour displacement of the ionic charge to the C-3 site; it would also tend to favour electrostatically less repulsing forms in which the double bond would be lost as a result of uptake of H and OH by the two carbons, or a follow-up of a Cannizaro-like auto-oxidation/reduction activity catalysed by complex formation with multivalent cations.

1.3.2. Types of physicochemical interactions of the ascorbate ion or of ascorbic acid

Several types of physicochemical interactions can be visualized:

H... bonded associations. These have been considered in section 1.2.8.

Electrostatic. These comprise associations of ascorbate ion with a cation such as guanidinium (intrinsically involving H... bonding) or complexing with a metal cation. Both these types have been considered in sections 1.2.7 and 1.2.8.

Hydrophilic associations. The ascorbate and ascorbic acid entities have several hydrophilic loci, namely the charged group itself or its hydroxyl forerunner, and the free OH groups present on C-5 and C-6. H... bonded association of water with the carbonyl group (C-1)=O can also be expected.

Hydrophobic trends. Examination of the molecular model in Fig. 1.1 shows a hydrophobic area which is composed of adjoining CH groups. As pointed out in section 1.2.6, the planar ring structure itself is expected to display hydrophobic-like effects by adversely affecting 3-dimensional water-structures.

The hydrophobically enforced water structures adjoining the free hydrophobic areas of the ascorbic/ascorbate entities can be diagrammatically represented as:

See also Lewin, 1974a.

Water-mediated hydrophobic/hydrophilic links. As pointed out elsewhere (Lewin, 1974a) the entropy change of water extrusion can act as a driving force for hydrophobic adherence, for H... bonded associations, and also for the attainment of water-mediated hydrophobic-hydrophilic group associations, thus

1.3.3. Oxidation-reduction and electron-transfer activities

1.3.3.1. *General*

Oxidation can be expressed in terms of loss of electrons as well as in terms of loss of hydrogen. Thus, the oxidation of ascorbate to dehydroascorbate can be expressed as proceeding via the loss of an electron to form the ascorbate free radical followed by further loss of 1 electron and 1 H^+ to form dehydroascorbic, as shown in Fig. 1.4.

It is generally considered that because the standard redox potential (E_0) of the thiol-disulphide system is well below that of the ascorbate/dehydroascorbic system, the former reduces DHA to AA. This evaluation is correct under standard conditions. However, the redox potential is a logarithmic function of the concentrations of the reduced and oxidized states, thus

$$E_h = E_0 - \frac{RT}{nF} \ln\{ [ox] / [red] \}$$ (1.7)

where E_h is the redox potential of the system, R is the gas constant, n is the number of electrons lost in the formation of the oxidized form (ox) from the reduced form (red), and F is the Faraday constant.

When the ratio of {(ascorbate)/(dehydroascorbic)} is very high, say $>10^4$, assisted by a high concentration ratio {$(-S-S-)/(-SH)^2$} —say 10^5, see Table 2.2—the ascorbate system should be capable of reducing a proportion of the disulphide present to its thiol counterpart.

1.3.3.2. *Electron-transfer activities*

The reaction of ascorbic acid with nicotinamide. The mixing of a solution containing nicotinamide with one containing ascorbic acid results instantaneously in the production of a yellow colour which has been interpreted as being due to complex formation (Milhorat, 1944). The reaction was shown to involve a 1:1 stoichiometry by Bailey *et al.* (1945). Najer and Guepet (1954) using spectroscopy concluded that the isolated product was primarily an ascorbate-nicotinamide salt, but that the reaction involved some association between the amide group and a secondary hydroxyl group of the acid. Guttman and Brooke (1963) concluded that the 1:1 stoichiometric complex consisted of {(ascorbate anion)—(protonated nicotinamide)} the optimum formation of which takes place at pH 3.8 with a standard enthalpy change of −1.5 kcal.

Nicotinamide derivatives, such as NAD, can reasonably be expected to form such complexes. This inference is lent support by the findings of Schneider and Staudinger (1965); see also section 2.3.2.2.

Reduction of aminochromes by ascorbic acid. Ascorbic acid reduces aminochromes. The oxidation-reduction has been formulated as proceeding via the free radicals of both reactants. In the case of adrenochrome interaction with ascorbic acid, the final products comprise 5:6 dihydroxy-N-methylindole and DHA. The reaction is considered in further detail in section 2.2.5.

1.3.4. Reactivity and reactions of the ascorbate anion

1.3.4.1. *Reactivity*

The various reactions of the ascorbate anion in forming a complex with metal ions and its other activities have already been noted in sections 1.2.6, 1.2.7 and 1.3.3. Reactivity in respect of oxidation/reduction can be significantly influenced by association of the ascorbate anion (and of ascorbic acid), via their hydrophobic areas, with the hydrophobic areas of other compounds, such as proteins, when the ionizable double-bond section of the ascorbic entity is free. This is so because the reactivity of the ionizable double-bond section of the ring is bound to be affected by the surrounding water-structures. The latter are effectively influenced by the proximity of the hydrophobic areas. By decreasing the influence of the hydro-phobically enforced water-structures (see Lewin, 1974a), the active section of the ascorbate is freer to undergo reaction. In other words, that part of the energy of activation enforced by the higher extent of structuring of water (which has to be overcome for reactivity) no longer opposes ionization. See also section 1.2.5.2 and Chapter 3 where the behaviour of 3′-5′cyclic AMP phosphodiesterase as ascorbate-lactonase is considered in detail.

1.3.4.2. *Reaction with histamine*

Ascorbate possesses a resonance activity between the C-2 and the C-3 sites. The iminazolium group of histamine also possesses a

$$H_2N-CH_2-CH_2-\overset{5}{C}\!=\!=\!=\!\overset{1}{CH}$$

$$HN\underset{4}{\overset{}{\diagdown}}\!\leftarrow\!\oplus\!\rightarrow\!\overset{2}{NH}$$

$$\underset{H}{\overset{|}{C}}\,3$$

potential for resonance which involves the two nitrogen sites. Since a cation with a resonance potential should tend to be associated with an anion with a resonance potential, the probability of association between the histamine cation and ascorbate should be significant. Further, from molecular model construction, it can be shown that a number of associations are feasible, one of which involves H... acceptance by the terminal amino group of histamine from the (C-3)OH group of ascorbate, accompanied by H... donation from (N-4)H of histamine to the (C-2)O⁻ group of ascorbate (see Fig. 1.8). These considerations prompted me to search for spectrophotometric evidence for association/interaction between ascorbate and hist-amine; the result was positive.*

---

* It is relevant to note that Edlbacher and Segesser (1937) observed that ascorbate, in presence of traces of ferric sulphate and exerted a destructive influence on histidine and on other molecules containing iminazole.

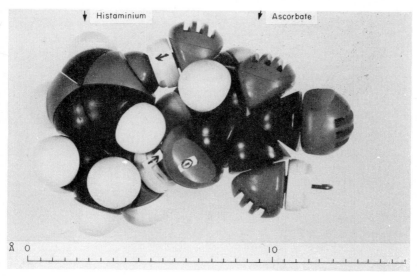

Fig. 1.8. Photograph of a correctly proportioned space-filling molecular model (constructed from CPK atomic models) of a stereochemically and energetically admissible complex of the cation of histamine with the anion of ascorbic acid.

As the reaction was time-dependent, since only *dilute* ascorbate solutions could be employed spectrophotometrically, and as high ionic strength had to be avoided in order to inhibit interference with the ionic nature of the histamine-ascorbate interaction, EDTA addition proved useful in removing multivalent cationic interference. The reaction displayed somewhat different characteristics depending on whether EDTA was present or not. In presence of EDTA, under anaerobic conditions and careful restriction of light, histamine was found to cause significant hypochromicity in the absorption spectrum of ascorbate. See Fig. 1.9. If light was not excluded, and also in the absence of EDTA, the histamine contribution to the ascorbate/histamine optical absorbance soon disappeared. From this one may infer that AFR is inimical to histamine.

1.3.4.3. *Reaction with nitrites and nitrosamines*

The reaction of ascorbate with nitrite results in the formation of nitric oxide and some nitrous oxide and nitrogen. The kinetics of the interaction show clear dependence on pH in the range of 0 to 4 (Dahn *et al.*, 1960; Evans and McAuliffe, 1956; Walters and Taylor,

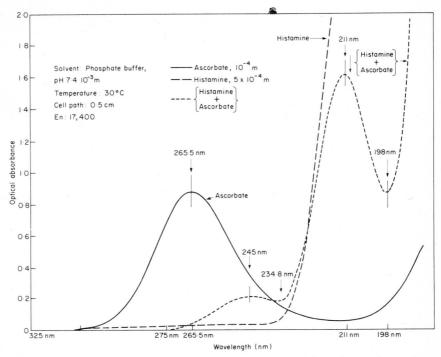

Fig. 1.9. Optical changes in the reaction between histamine and ascorbate. Optical recordings carried out on a calibrated PE-450 spectrophotometer using continuous purging with N_2 free from O_2 and CO_2, and using a 0.5 cm optical path length. All measurements were carried out in an atmosphere of N_2 free from O_2 and CO_2. 30°C $\epsilon_{(265.5, ascorbate)} = 17,400$. Solvent: 10^{-3} M phosphate buffer, pH 7.4. Anaerobic conditions. Histamine = 5×10^{-4} M. Measurements were carried out within two to four hours of preparation of the solutions.

1964) and it was considered that the ascorbate/nitrite complex formed would break down to give "monodehydroascorbic acid" i.e. AFR. It has been observed that the ascorbate anion is nitrosated 240 times as fast as the ascorbic acid (Mirvish *et al.*, 1972). For biological activity of ascorbate in respect of inhibition of nitrosamine formation see section 4.8.3.

1.3.5. The monodehydroascorbate free radical (AFR) (see also sections 1.2.4.1 and 1.2.4.2)

1.3.5.1. *Existence and formulation*

Originally the oxidation of vitamin C by oxygen was considered to lead directly to the dehydroascorbic entity. However, Bezssonoff and

Wolosyn (1938) advanced experimental evidence in favour of the formation of an intermediate product having the formula $C_6H_7O_6$. This intermediate form was originally termed monodehydroascorbic acid or monodehydroascorbate. Weissenberger and Luvalle (1944) visualized the existence of a semiquinone free radical as an intermediate in the mechanism of the copper catalysis of the oxidation of ascorbic acid.

The existence of this semiquinone-like free radical has been established by ESR measurements (e.g. Yamazaki *et al.*, 1959, 1960, 1961, 1962). The position of the unpaired electron has been subject to argument. One school of thought views it as an ascorbate free radical (e.g. Lagercrantz, 1964; Duke, 1968; Russel *et al.*, 1966), and allocates it to the O on the C-2 position, thus

$$
\begin{array}{c}
CH_2OH \\
| \\
HOCH \\
| \\
HC\!-\!O\!-\!C\!=\!O \\
| \qquad | \\
C\!=\!C \\
| \qquad | \\
\underline{O} \qquad O^{\cdot}
\end{array}
$$

while others (e.g. Foerster *et al.*, 1965) view it as an ascorbic *acid* free radical and allocate the unpaired electron to the oxygen on the C-3 site, thus

$$
\begin{array}{c}
CH_2OH \\
| \\
HOCH \\
| \\
HC\!-\!O\!-\!C\!=\!O \\
| \qquad | \\
C\!=\!C \\
| \qquad | \\
O^{\cdot} \qquad O \\
\qquad \quad | \\
\qquad \quad H
\end{array}
$$

It is possible that the unpaired electron of the AFR formed at acid pH values is located at the C-3 site, while that formed in the alkaline pH range is located at the C-2 site. However, the available data appear insufficient to decide on the locations unequivocally. AFR has been characterized by Levandowski *et al.* (1964). Complexing with ascorbic acid was also indicated. See also Kluge *et al.* (1967).

1.3.5.2. *Formation and removal*

The concentration of the AFR at a given time depends on its rate of formation and of disappearance. It can be formed in several types of reactions and eliminated in others; an overall view of these is as follows:

Formation	Method	Elimination

(a) Mixing of AA with DHA resulting in equilibrium

(b) Oxidation of AA with molecular oxygen

(c) Reaction of AA with oxidants

(d) Irradiation with light

Non-enzymatic

(e) Enzymatic redox reactions involving AA

Enzymatic

(a) Dismutation into AA and DHA

(b) Transformation into AA by capturing an electron or an H atom from another substance (and thereby causing the latter to become a free radical)

(c) Enzymatic redox reactions

These will now be outlined in turn:

1.3.5.3. *Formation of AFR*

Mixing of AA with DHA. The mixing of AA and DHA in acid pH ranges has been shown by Foerster *et al.* (1965) to yield the ascorbic free radical. They computed an equilibrium constant value of *c.* 5×10^{-9} at pH 6.4 and 25°C. Decrease in pH was found to result in decreased equilibrium constant values, from 5.1×10^{-9} at pH 6.4 to 5.6×10^{-12} at pH 4.0. The reversible reaction was formulated as

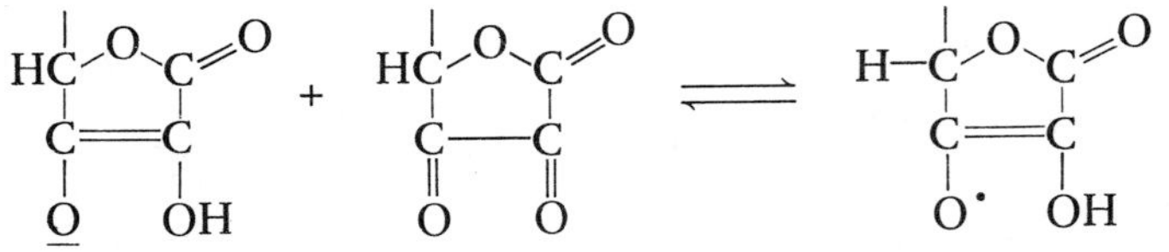

$$\text{Ascorbate} + \text{DHA} \rightleftharpoons \text{AFR} \tag{1.8}$$

from which the equlibrium constant was formulated as

$$\frac{[\text{AFR}]^2}{[\text{AA}^-][\text{DHA}]} = \text{K} \tag{1.9}$$

Balancing of the reaction is however more precise in terms of ascorbic acid thus

$$+ \ H^+ \longrightarrow \qquad\qquad\qquad (1.10)$$

Ascorbate free radical   Ascorbic acid
                                free radical

$$\qquad\qquad\qquad\qquad\qquad\qquad (1.11)$$

DHA   Ascorbic acid

The latter formation may be visualized as proceeding via the intermediate formation of a double-H... bonded ascorbic acid:DHA complex which would tend to be formed more readily with increasing acidity, thus

It will be appreciated that the concentration of the free radical is very small under the given conditions. However, as is the case in many other reactions, infeed of energy—such as that emanating from an exergonic reaction—can result in much higher, albeit transient, concentrations of AFR.

Oxidation with molecular oxygen. Lagercrantz (1964) detected the formation of AFR in ascorbate solutions containing dissolved oxygen, in the pH range of 6.6 to 9.6. The ESR spectrum of the free radical was observed for several hours when the tubes containing the solutions were stoppered.

The *two step* oxidation of ascorbic acid has been demonstrated by Blois (1958) on titration with the stable free radical diphenylpicrylhydrazyl, thus

$$[DPPH]^{\bullet} + AAHH \rightarrow [DPPH_2] + [AAH]^{\bullet}$$

$$[DPPH]^{\bullet} + [AAH]^{\bullet} \rightarrow [DPPH_2] + DHA$$

This process is an example of "scavenging" of free radicals by ascorbic acid.

Irradiation with light. As noted earlier in this chapter, ascorbate solutions on being subjected to normal, diffuse, daylight undergo deactivation, which can be attributed to initial formation of free radicals. The formation of ascorbate/bic free radicals can be reasonably postulated, thus

$$AA^- + h^v \rightarrow AFR^-$$

The significance of the ability of EDTA and other chelating/complexing agents to offset deactivation of ascorbate by daylight can be understood as follows:

The formation of an ascorbate free radical from ascorbate requires the ejection of an electron. Irradiation of the ascorbate solution with very short UV light or X-rays can supply the necessary energy. When however only longer wavelengths are available—e.g. diffuse daylight—the energy supplied by irradiation falls short of the minimum required. The balance of energy required for the electron-ejection can be met by coupling the electron-ejection process to an electron-capturing process such as is available in oxidation-reduction reactions e.g. in

$$Fe^{+++} + e \rightarrow Fe^{++}$$

We then have for the overall reaction

$$AA^- + h^v + Fe^{+++} \rightarrow AFR^- + Fe^{++}$$

See also page 34.

Enzymatic redox reactions involving AA⁻. These are considered in section 2.3.2.

1.3.5.4. *Removal of AFR*

Dismutation into AA and DHA. This can be formulated in terms of equations (1.10) and (1.11) as in section 1.3.5.2.

Transformation into AA/AA⁻ by capturing an electron or an H atom from another substance, thereby causing the latter to become a free radical. The reaction can be represented as

$$AFR + X \rightarrow AA + X^•$$

where $X^•$ is the free radical form of X.

Such a mechanism has been proposed by Blumberg *et al.* (1965) in the enzymatic β-hydroxylation of DOPA to noradrenaline, where AFR reacts with dopamine to produce a dopamine free-radical. See also section 2.3.2.4.

Enzymatic redox reactions. Enzymatic redox reactions have been shown to produce ascorbate/bic free radicals. For a review and re-interpretations see section 2.3.

1.3.5.5. *Other non-enzymatic reactions involving the ascorbic/ate free radical*

AFR has been implicated in several reactions. One that is of interest regarding the biological role of ascorbic acid (see section 4.3.2) lies in the reaction with adrenochrome. Adrenochrome is known to be reduced by ascorbic acid resulting in the formation of 5,6-dihydroxyindole and DHA. It has been found possible to give a satisfactory interpretation of the kinetics of the reaction in terms involving both the free radical of ascorbic acid and the free radical of adrenochrome* (Mattok, 1965). The overall scheme comprising both free radicals is presented on page 34. (For a review of reduction of adrenochrome, see Heacock and Powell, 1973.)

1.3.5.6. *Reactivity*

Semiquinone-like free-radicals possess a significant energy (above that of the precursor) which can be contributed to the lowering of the energy of activation of an associated reaction. Take, for instance, a reaction involving ascorbic acid (or ascorbate)—not necessarily an oxidation-reaction—such as

$$\text{Ascorbate} + X \rightarrow \text{Ascorbate} - X \rightarrow \text{Ascorbate} + Y$$

which involves a comparatively high energy of activation. This in itself need not form a free-radical. However, slight oxidation of the ascorbate by an appropriate oxidizing agent—which results in the intermediate formation of the free-radical—should speed up the above reaction significantly. See also section 2.3.2.

---

* Evidence for the existence of an adrenochrome free radical was obtained by Borg (1965).

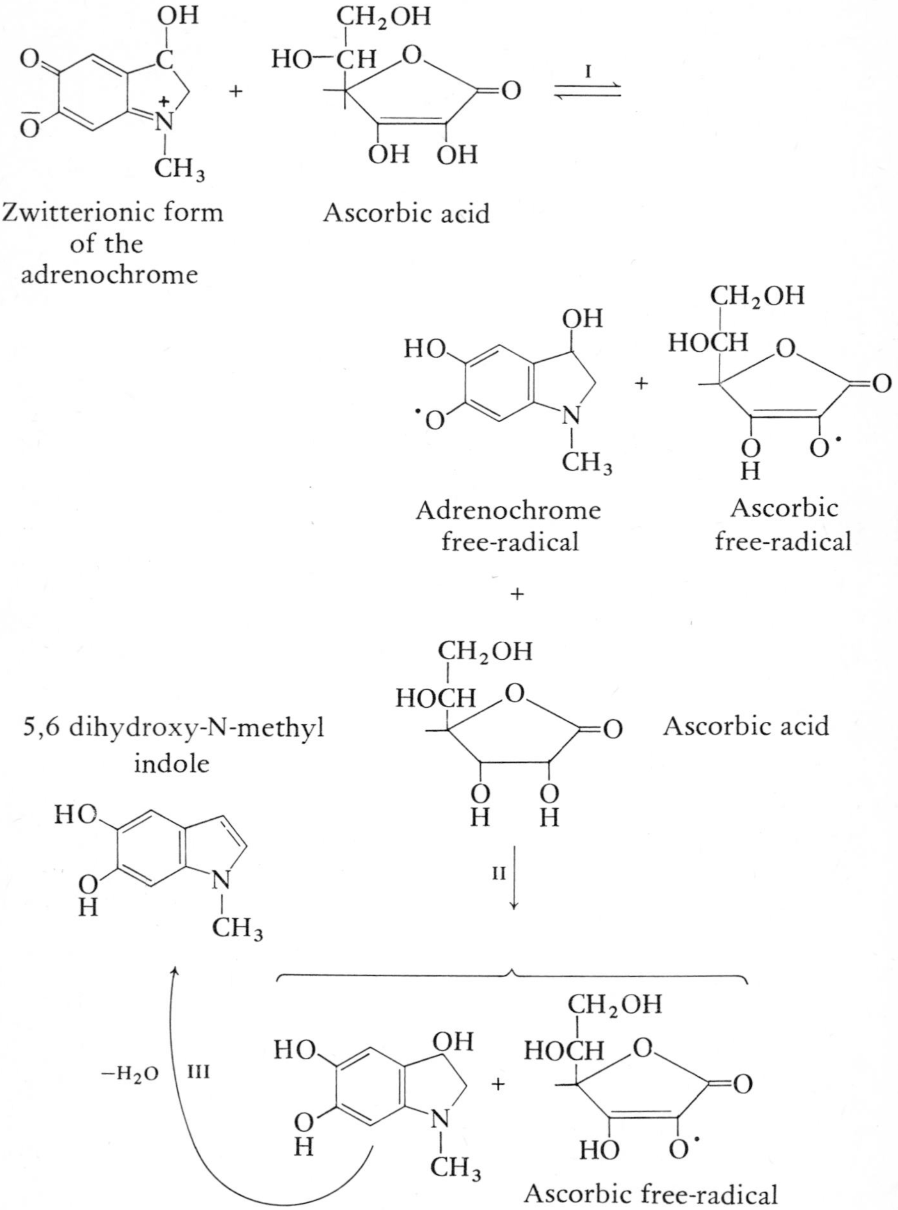

Zwitterionic form
of the
adrenochrome

Ascorbic acid

Adrenochrome
free-radical

Ascorbic
free-radical

5,6 dihydroxy-N-methyl
indole

Ascorbic acid

$-H_2O$ III

Ascorbic free-radical

2 Ascorbic free-radicals $\xrightarrow{\text{IV}}$ DHA + Ascorbic *acid*

1.3.5.7. *Ascorbate/bic free radical involvement with water free-radicals*

In reviewing the various factors concerned with ascorbate insta-bility, it was found helpful to invoke the existence of water free-radicals, that is of a water molecule containing a single, unpaired electron, thus

H_2O^+, which can be represented diagrammatically as H:Ö:
                                                          ̤
                                                          H

Compare this with the other ionic forms of water:

$$\text{H}_3\text{O}^+, \quad \text{i.e.} \quad \text{H:Ö:} , \quad \text{and} \quad \text{H}_2\text{O}, \quad \text{i.e.} \quad \text{H:Ö:}$$

This concept enables collation of the destabilizing of ascorbate by (i) the presence of multivalent cations, (ii) increasing dilution in water, and (iii) photosensitivity. The overall scheme comprises the existence (albeit cation-attached and transient) of a water free-radical and of the two forms of the ascorbic/bate free-radical, namely

Ascorbic free-radical   Ascorbate free-radical

in terms of the following (see Lewin, 1975a).

Electron donor/acceptor trends. A negatively charged resonating free radical should have a greater electron-donor trend than the non-charged form of the free radical. Hence the ascorbate form of the free radical should be a more potent electron-donor than the ascorbic form.

In comparing Fe^{++} and Fe^{+++} forms of the iron cation, Fe^{+++} should have the greater electron-acceptor trend, while Fe^{++} should have a greater electron-donor trend. Thus, the preferred associations in electron-donor and electron-acceptor involvements should be $\{[Fe^{3+}] [\text{Ascorbate free-radical}]\}$, and $\{[Fe^{2+}] [\text{Ascorbic free-radical}]\}$.

Representation of the hexahydrated redox system including a water free-radical. The redox system of the hexahydrated iron cations is usually represented as

$$[Fe^{++} \cdot 6H_2O] \xrightleftharpoons[+e]{-e} [Fe^{3+} \cdot 6H_2O]$$

It is advocated here that the ferric ion, because of its higher electron-pulling trend, can exist in an equilibrium with an associated H_2O^+ free-radical, thus

$$\left[\begin{array}{c} 5H_2O \cdot Fe^{3+} \\ \ddot{Q}\!:\!H \end{array} \right]^{3+*} \xrightleftharpoons \left[\begin{array}{c} 5H_2O \cdot Fe^{2+} \\ H \overset{..}{\underset{..}{O}}\!\!\overset{H}{\underset{+}{}} \end{array} \right]^{3+}$$

$$\text{I} \qquad\qquad\qquad\qquad \text{II}$$

The tendency for transient existence of the water free-radical (within form II) should increase when an ascorbate free-radical is electrically attracted to the hydrated ferric ion, thus

Hydrated Fe^{3+} ion   Ascorbate free-radical

The latter complex undergoes a loss of the unpaired electron on the constituent ascorbate free-radical to the ferric ion, accompanied by bond rearrangements to give DHA, thus

Hydrated Fe^{2+} ion   Dehydroascorbic entity

---

* The arrows associated with the electrons to the H_2O molecule show their tendency to be displaced. One electron of the lone-pair of the oxygen adjacent to the Fe^{3+} would be attracted to the positive anhydrous core; an electron from the second lone-pair would then tend to be displaced as shown, thereby tending partially to compensate for the change.

In contrast with the ferric ion, the hydrated ferrous ion is capable of losing an electron to the ascor*bic* free-radical (followed by rearrangement to a ferric ion and ascorbate anion) thus

Hydrated Fe^{2+} ion   Ascorbic free-radical

Hydrated Fe^{3+} ion   Ascorbate anion

Thus, the Fe^{2+}/Fe^{3+} redox system can use an ascorbate free-radical and an ascorbic free-radical to oxidize/reduce them to DHA (which breaks down readily) and ascorbate. The inactivation of the ascorbate system can thus be understood to depend on the initial production of ascorbic/ate free-radicals following exposure to light, in agreement with findings previously noted in this chapter.

1.3.6. The dehydroascorbic entity (DHA)

1.3.6.1. *Formation and formulation*

DHA is formed by oxidation of ascorbic acid/ascorbate, as illustrated in Fig. 1.4. Several laboratory preparations have been described, e.g. Pecherer (1951), and Patterson (1950). The anhydrous form is unable to act as an acid because it lacks ionizable OH groups on the lactone ring. However, it does exhibit acid ionization with a pK value of *c.* 9 (Borsook *et al.*, 1937). This acidity can be met by hydration of the carbonyl groups at sites C-2 and C-3 as illustrated in Fig. 1.4 (see also Roe, 1954; Raiha, 1958). Such hydration is also likely to reduce effectively the considerable electrostatic repulsion between the negative ends of the carbonylic dipoles. On this basis, it is generally accepted that DHA exists also in the hydrated form—probably predominantly—although the relative portions of the various species have not been ascertained.

1.3.6.2. *Reactivity*

DHA is considered to be highly unstable in aqueous solution because it is highly reactive, easily reduced and because its ring structure is easily ruptured by hydrolysis to give 2-3:diketogluconic acid which is a more potent reducing agent than ascorbic acid (Borsook *et al.*, 1937).

Interaction with thiol groups: DHA reacts with an —SH group containing compounds such as cysteine, glutathione and thioglycollic acid. Two steps have been recognized in the overall reaction:

(i) A stoichiometric 1:1 complex formation which can be represented as

$$R-SH + O=C \overset{\frown}{\underset{\smile}{(DHA)}} \longrightarrow$$

The formation of these compounds was established by Drake *et al.* (1942) using optical rotation and iodine titrations.

The overall reaction can be considered as an oxidation-reduction reaction, thus

$$2\ R-SH + 2\ DHA \rightarrow R-S-S-R + 2AA$$

Interaction with amino/imino groups: Because the anhydrous form possesses active carbonyl groups, it can react with amino/imino groups, thus

The amino group of dinitrophenylhydrazine reacts with the carbonyl groups of DHA with water elimination. The reaction is widely used for the assay of DHA. (For numerous references and reviews see Roe (1954-5, 1961) and Roe and Kuether (1943)).

1.3.7. L-ascorbic-2-sulphate

L-ascorbic-2-sulphate (AAS) has been found in the urine of humans and other animals including rats and fish. It is itself biologically inactive, but has attracted much interest because of the possibility that tracing of its metabolic origin would lead to further elucidation of AA metabolism. Tolbert *et al.* (1975) and Seale (1973) give details of the preparation of the substance.

Verlangieri and Mumma (1973) obtained evidence that cholestrol is sulphated *in vivo* by L-ascorbic sulphate.

1.3.8. Ascorbic phosphates

Several L-ascorbic phosphates have been prepared by Nomura *et al.*; further details are given by Tolbert *et al.* (1974, 1975). The biological significance of these entities is under investigation.

Chapter 2

Biochemical reactivity

2.1. Apportionment of biochemical reactivity to the ascorbic, mono-dehydroascorbic (AFR) and dehydroascorbic entities

2.1.1. Individual contributions

AA, AFR and DHA are known to participate in biochemical reactions, AA as a reducing agent, AFR both as a reducing agent and as an oxidizing agent as appropriate, and DHA as an oxidizing agent as well as an entity combining with groups containing labile hydrogens (i.e. $-SH$, $-NH_2$ or $-NH$). As the mixing of AA and DHA results in formation of very small quantities of AFR (Foerster et al., 1965) any differentiation would appear to be correspondingly blurred. However, while there is clear evidence that AFR can be formed both enzymatically and non-enzymatically (e.g. Yamazaki and Piette, 1961; Ohnishi et al., 1969; see also section 1.3.5) there does not seem to be evidence that the reduction of DHA proceeds via AFR. Further, the activity of each entity can be delineated in a number of areas; and overall appreciation of the numerous activities of the AA/AFR/DHA system should be assisted by recognition of individual trends as distinct from interconvertibility.

AA and DHA can be viewed as antagonists, since their activities follow opposing directions. Further, AA, under physiological conditions, displays an ionic character, whereas DHA is more hydrophobic in character. Thus, at neutral pH values, AA (pK $\sim$ 4.18) is an anion, while DHA (pK $\sim$ 9) is hardly ionized. Indeed, the anhydrous form of DHA displays its relatively non-ionic character by being more lipid-soluble as indicated by the respective distribution coefficients of DHA and AA in butanol at pH 7.4, namely 0.1 and

40

0.01 (Martin, 1961). Following this experimental trend has led a number of investigators to conclude that DHA penetrates lipid membranes, such as those of erythrocytes (e.g. Lloyd, 1951; Christine *et al.*, 1956) and of brain (Patterson and Mastin, 1951), more readily than AA. Indeed, the penetration of lipid membranes by DHA is in line with the possession of three carbonyl groups in one plane, and with the associated expectation that it should reduce the interfacial tension to a greater extent than AA (Lewin, 1974a).

2.1.2. Individual stabilities

The individual stabilities of the three ascorbic entities obviously affect their respective contributions. It has already been pointed out that at low ionic strength the free ascorbate ion is comparatively unstable. Now the concentration of ascorbate in individuals well supplied with vitamin C is of the order of 1 mg to 2 mg per 100 ml of plasma, i.e. $c.$ 5×10^{-5} M to 10^{-4} M. In absence of stabilizing agents the ascorbate should be rapidly deactivated. However, plasma is approximately 0.8% NaCl in content, i.e. $c.$ 2×10^{-1} M NaCl. From what has been stated earlier (see sections 1.2.1 and 1.2.5) the ascorbate should be afforded some protection by such ionic strength. Additional protection is likely to be afforded by several proteins which associate with ascorbate.

The stability of DHA is restricted by its ability to undergo hydrolytic ring rupture (i.e. de-lactonization), to 2:3-diketogulonic acid and further on, by oxidation, to 1-threonic acid, as well as by re-convertibility to ascorbate by reduced glutathione and other —SH groups. It is well known that DHA is unstable in alkaline solution (e.g. Borsook *et al.*, 1937); the instability can be ascribed to the considerable electrostatic-polar repulsion within the negatively charged ion. Instability in the acid pH region below pH 4 in biochemical media has been documented (Hughes and Maton, 1968).

The biochemical reactivity of AFR can be viewed in terms of its ability to act as an oxidant or as a reductant in appropriate redox systems. However, its oxidizing ability to remove a single electron from several biochemical compounds and thereby turn them into free-radicals clearly gives it a significance which deserves emphasis. Indeed, it is this characteristic which probably enables the ascorbate system to participate effectively in several well-known enzymatic hydroxylating reactions—such as the formation of noradrenaline from dopamine and that of tryptamine from tryptophan. These hydroxylations will be considered in sections 2.3.2.4 and 2.3.2.5.

2.2. Reducing properties of ascorbate and of the ascorbic free-radical

The ability of the ascorbic/dehydroascorbic system to participate in biochemical oxidation/reductions is well known; the literature uses the standard redox emfs, determined under *equilibrium conditions*, for evaluation of the direction of spontaneous oxidation or reduction. The principle is sound provided simple systems are used, all the components are known, and the possibility of infeed of energy can be excluded. However, biochemical systems are mostly complex, and they also comprise *steady state* concentrations of the AFR which result from associated energy-infeed processes. Hence, relevant conclusions as to the direction of oxidation or reduction based on thermodynamic *equilibrium* conditions may well prove to be invalid. As computation of the direction of reaction in biochemical systems is of fundamental importance, I shall first outline current principles and their utilization for computing the probable direction of oxidation/reduction in the interaction of the ascorbic/dehydroascorbic system with the thiol/disulphide system. This will be followed by consideration of the effect of energy-infeed from associated reactions resulting in the presence of *excess* AFR concentrations (i.e. in steady state concentrations of AFR which are much higher than those found under *equilibrium* conditions). It is relevant to draw attention here to the repeated observations that—in physiological malfunctions—low thiol concentrations exist along with low ascorbate concentrations (e.g. Heath, 1962; Dische and Zill, 1951). Elevation of ascorbate content of tissue by mega intake of ascorbic acid tends to raise tissue −SH content (and inhibit the malfunction) thereby indicating that ascorbate contributes to reduction of disulphides. This indication is supported by findings in which sulphydryl reducing agents can be satisfactorily replaced by ascorbate (e.g. Price, 1966). Such phenomena are at first sight difficult to comprehend on the basis of thermodynamic equilibrium conditions, but can be understood in terms of the relationships developed here.

The potential of the ascorbate system to induce higher ratios of {[thiol]/[disulphide]} than those expected on the basis of thermodynamic equilibrium conditions, can be enhanced by

(a) *Increase in ability to reduce disulphides.* This can be conveniently discussed under

(i) Formation by associated enzymatic reactions of the ascorbic free-radical in steady state concentrations much higher than equilibrium values *and* in energetically higher states (i.e. electronically excited states).

(ii) A more negative value of the redox potential of the ascorbate/dehydroascorbate system following reduction in exposed area of hydrophobic groups on their adherence.

(b) *Ability to reduce, or combine with, thiol group oxidants.* This is exemplified by the reduction of adrenochrome by the ascorbic system.

Enhancement due to these reactions will be considered in the following sections.

2.2.1. Utilization of redox potentials in evaluation of reducing trends

The ability of the ascorbic system to reduce other biochemical entities can be evaluated in terms of the respective redox potentials. Calculations utilizing this approach can involve errors unless care is taken to specify the direction of reaction and the relevant mathematical signs. Hence it is desirable to give more than a bare outline.

In employing redox relations it is essential to state whether they express oxidation or reduction. The process

$$\text{Oxidant} \xrightarrow{+ne} \text{Reductant}$$

(where "n" is the number of electrons involved) finds expression in the redox relation

$$E_{h\,\text{(oxidation)}} = E'_{0\,\text{(oxidation)}} + \frac{RT}{nF} \ln \{\,[\text{oxidant}]\,/\,[\text{reductant}]\,\} \qquad (2.1)$$

where E_h is the redox potential of the system, E'_0 is the relevant *standard* redox potential (i.e. when the ratio $\{[\text{oxidant}]/[\text{reductant}]\}$ is unity) under the given conditions, R is the gas constant, T is the Absolute Temperature, and F is the Faraday (i.e. 96,500 coulombs), and where the respective activities are equated with their concentrations.

The free energy change of a redox reaction can be written in the form

$$\Delta G = -nFE_h \qquad (2.2a)$$

Where standard conditions apply—namely when the activities of the reactants and products are each unity—we have

$$\Delta G^\circ = -nFE'_0 \qquad (2.2b)$$

When two reactions are linked, the spontaneous direction of the combined reaction can be predicted using the principle that for spontaneity the sum-total of the free energies must be negative; thus for the combination of reactions I and II

$$\Delta G = \Delta G_I + \Delta G_{II} \tag{2.3}$$

and

$$\{\Delta G_I + \Delta G_{II}\} < 0 \tag{2.4}$$

Hence,

$$\{-nF(E_I + E_{II})\} < 0 \quad (2.5a), \quad \text{or} \quad \{E_I + E_{II}\} > 0 \tag{2.5b}$$

2.2.2. Conditions favouring reduction of disulphides

Using the respective standard redox potentials let us now evaluate the conditions under which the ascorbic/dehydroascorbic system can reduce the thiol/disulphide system, under equilibrium conditions. In Table 2.1 are given the redox potential values for different systems under the specified conditions.

Table 2.1. Redox potential values of the ascorbic system and some thiol/disulphide systems. (All values are for *reduction* processes)

System	Standard Redox EMF	pH	$T^{\circ}C$
DHA → AA	+0.058	7.0	25–30
Cystine → Cysteine	−0.33	7.0	25
Glutathione (oxid. → red.)	−0.33*	7.0	25
Thiolactic acid (oxid. → red.)	−0.32	7.0	30
Dithiothreitol (oxid. → red.)	−0.332	7.0	30
Dithiothreitol (oxid. → red.)	−0.336	8.1	30

* Different investigators give different values for the standard redox potentials of individual −SH/−S−S− systems. The variations depend to some extent on the methods used for the calculations. The value of −0.33 volts quoted here is favoured by several investigators, although the value of −0.23 has also been given.

To ascertain whether the reaction

$$2 R—SH + DHA \rightleftharpoons R—S—S—R + AA \tag{2.6}$$

proceeds to the right or to the left—i.e. whether thiol will reduce DHA to AA, or whether AA will be oxidized to DHA while reducing the disulphide to thiol—we have to decide whether the forward or the reverse reaction will result in an overall positive redox emf.

The overall process results from linking of the following two reactions

$$AA \rightleftharpoons DHA + 2e + 2H^+ \qquad (I)$$
$$-S-S- + 2H^+ + 2e \rightleftharpoons 2 -SH \qquad (II)$$

The forward process is associated with $_I E'_{0(oxidation)} = -0.058$ and $_{II} E'_{0(reduction)} = -0.33$, thus resulting in a *combined* $E'_0 = -0.388$. Hence the forward reaction is non-spontaneous.

For the reverse reaction—in which the $-SH/-S-S-$ system is oxidized, while the DHA/AA system is reduced—we have

$$\begin{array}{l} _I E'_{0\,(reduction)} = +0.058 \\ _{II} E'_{0\,(oxidation)} = +0.33 \end{array} \rightarrow Combined\ E'_0 = +0.388$$

Hence, the mixing of the $-SH/-S-S-$ system and the ascorbate system each in unit activities will result in reduction of DHA to AA, accompanied by oxidation of 2 $-SH$ to $-S-S-$.

The respective values of the redox potentials of the two systems vary with the respective concentrations of the individual oxidants and reductants. It is necessary therefore to determine whether changes in such concentrations can tilt the balance in favour of the AA/DHA system reducing the $-S-S-/-SH$ system. Relation 2.1 can be used to this end. The computed results are plotted in Fig. 2.1.* Inspection of the figure shows that high concentration ratio of $\{[AA]/[DHA]\}$ such as over 10^3 should be capable of reducing high $\{[sulphide]/[sulphydryl]\}$ concentration ratios of c. 10^{16} and over.

It is worthwhile pondering that in a system in which the DHA formed is rapidly removed, ascorbate reduction of the disulphide can proceed effectively despite the constraints imposed thermo-dynamically.

2.2.3. Effectiveness of the ascorbic free radical and of ascorbate as reducing agents for disulphides

Consider now the possibility of involvement of the ascorbate free radical AFR in reduction of disulphides. Three reducing activities

---

* This is based on the value of -0.33 for the reduction process $-S-S- \rightarrow 2 -SH$.

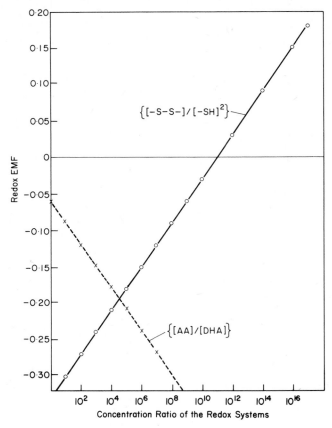

Fig. 2.1. Variation of the Redox E.M.F.s of the Disulphide/Thiol System and the Ascorbic System with the respective concentration ratios of the Redox Systems $(-S-S-)/(-SH)^2$ and $(AA)/(DHA)$.

may be visualized as a result of (a) oxidation of AA to AFR, (b) oxidation of AFR to DHA, and (c) the possession of high energy levels by nascent AFR molecules:

Linkage of the oxidation of AA to AFR to the reduction of disulphides.

$$2AA \rightarrow 2AFR + 2e + 2H^+$$

$$R-S-S-R + 2e + 2H^+ \rightarrow 2RSH$$

The value of $E_0' = +0.33^*$ for the AFR/AA system and hence -0.33 for AA $\rightarrow$ AFR, compares with that of the $-S-S- \rightarrow 2$-SH

---

* The value of 0.33 is the average of 0.34 (as given by Everling *et al.* (1969) and 0.32 obtained by Weis (1975)). See also section 1.2.4.2.

$(E'_0 = -0.33)$. The two systems should therefore be about at equilibrium under standard conditions. Thus formation of AFR increases the probability of disulphide being reduced.

Linkage of oxidation of AFR to DHA with reduction of disulphides.

$$2AFR \rightarrow DHA + 2e + 2H^+$$

$$R-S-S-R + 2e + 2H^+ \rightarrow 2RSH$$

No experimental value for the standard redox potential is available for the system AFR → DHA. Further it is believed, e.g. Nason *et al.* (1954), that DHA is reduced *directly* to AA; hence elucidation of this path should await evaluation of relevant data.

Linkage of nascent AFR activity to reduction of disulphides. The ability of reductants to reduce other molecular species increases when they are in an energetically higher state, such as that when the electrons are in an activated—or excited—state above that of normal. Highly activated states can be attained by various means. In general, a freshly formed entity is likely to be in an energetically higher state, because it is likely to possess—albeit transiently—part of the energy of the reaction.* Hence—at equal concentrations—a freshly formed AFR such as that formed by a co-existent reaction is likely to exercise a greater reducing power than a static, equilibrated AFR such as that present in an equilibrated mixture of AA, AFR and DHA. Further, the reducing *capacity* of a species depends not only on the energy level factor but also on the concentration of the species. Co-existence with a system which produces AFR concentrations several times greater than that of the static, equilibrated, state should therefore endow the ascorbic system with a greater reducing potency than that which involves only the static concentration of AFR. Numerous experimental observations can be integrated into this concept; it will be sufficient here to quote two:

(i) Ohnishi *et al.* (1969) observed that when ascorbate is added to a system containing horseradish peroxidase, p-cresol and H_2O_2, the ESR signal of monodehydro p-cresol (i.e. the free radical of p-cresol) is completely replaced by that of AFR, although ascorbate is a much slower substrate for peroxidase than p-cresol. Further, *the addition of 1 mM p-cresol caused a 16-fold increase in the rate of ascorbate oxidation, and a 46-fold increase in the steady state concentration of AFR.*

---

* A well known example is that of "nascent hydrogen" whose reducing power is very much greater than that of ordinary hydrogen; see also the Law of Formation of Non-Stable States (Lewin, 1974a).

(ii) Ascorbic acid oxidase can catalyse the reaction of substrates with which it does not react directly. Thus, the enzyme, in the presence of ascorbic acid, is able to reduce cytochrome c as a result of a secondary reaction in which AFR is formed (Yamazaki, 1962).

Although experimental data directly linking nascent AFR activity to the reduction of disulphides are not available, data are available which fit the suggestion that nascent AFR is capable of increasing the ratio $\{[SH]/[-S-S-]\}$. Thus ascorbate can replace sulphydryl groups (e.g. Price, 1966).

The decreased −SH and ascorbate concentration in ageing tissues (e.g. Dische and Zil, 1951), can be understood in terms in which the AFR produced is effectively mopped up by scavenging increased concentrations of free radicals and other substances, resulting in decreased ability to keep the $\{[-SH]/[S-S-]\}$ concentration ratios at the normal levels.

2.2.4. Hydrophobic effects on redox potential

Elsewhere (Lewin, 1974a) I have advanced the concept that the effect of increasing hydrophobic content in the reactant molecules and in the water-solvent medium can be expressed in terms of increased two-dimensional water-structuring at the expense of three-dimensional water-structuring of bulk-water. These changes have been computed to result in lowering of the interfacial tension and in decreased trends for acid dissociation because of the increased difficulty of abstracting individual water molecules from the bulk for ionization in the process

$$R-COOH + H_2O \rightleftharpoons RCOO^- + H_3O^+ \qquad (2.7)$$

We can express oxidation/reduction electron-loss/gain in parallel terms to those involved in acid ionization requirement of water, thus

$$AA^- \xrightarrow{\;+H_2O\;} H_2O^- + AFR \qquad (2.8)^*$$

$$2AFR + H_2O \rightarrow AAH + DHA \qquad (2.9)$$

On this basis the hydrophobically enforced two-dimensional structuring of bulk-water should favour *inhibition* of electron loss, i.e. the ability to be oxidized should be decreased. Conversely, the less hydrophobic the local situation is, the more readily should the

---

* The hydrated electron has been detected in liquid water during irradiation (Avery *et al.*, 1968; Likhtenstein, 1968).

system be oxidized, and the more negative (or less positive) should the redox potential become.

The increased negativity of the electrode potential can be expressed in relation (2.1) by making E_0' more negative and by assigning a higher value to the activity of the reductant.

Thus, decrease in hydrophobic content which makes oxidation of a reductant entity easier should correspondingly make the ascorbate reduction of disulphides easier. The reduction of exposed hydrophobic area can be attained by causing adherence between the hydrophobic segments of ascorbate with those of a suitable protein. A reduction in the proportion of (hydrophobic/hydrophilic) groups can be attained by increasing the proportion of {coil/helix} in a protein, since the process helix → coil at constant hydrophobic exposed area or at low content of hydrophobic adherence increases the proportion of (hydrophilic/hydrophobic) groups by liberating the hydrophilic groups C=O and NH from their H... bonding. Therefore we can expect that reduction of the hydrophobic areas resulting from hydrophobic adherence between ascorbate and a protein will result in increased tendency of ascorbate to reduce the disulphide group. Ascorbate-protein complexes have been detected in serum (e.g. Nichelmann et al., 1966; Fiddick and Heath, 1967) but the effect on the redox potential of the AA → DHA system has as yet not been experimentally determined.

2.2.5. Reduction of adrenochrome by ascorbic/ascorbate free-radical system

Ascorbate is capable of reducing various biochemical and organic compounds such as dichloro-phenolindophenol and adrenochrome. The reduction of adrenochrome involving AFR formation has already been noted in section 1.3.5.5. Because adrenochrome is a highly toxic substance which appears to act by virtue of its ability to combine with the −SH groups and finally convert them to disulphides [see also section 5.3.2], it is apposite to highlight the ascorbic activity in reduction of adrenochrome and associated inhibition of its toxic activity.

Reduced glutathione and enzymatic −SH groups are inactivated on association with carbonyl groups, often followed by their transformation into disulphides. The carbonyl groups of adrenochrome confer upon it the ability to deactivate −SH groups by interacting with them and eventually transforming them into disulphides.*

---

* For several references see the review by Heacock and Powell (1973).

However, if ascorbate is present it can reduce adrenochrome, thereby decreasing and even totally inhibiting the deactivation of −SH groups. The DHA formed as a result of the oxidation of AA is capable of oxidizing free −SH groups, but it can itself be deactivated by combination with free −NH$_2$ groups and by hydrolytic rupture of the lactone ring to 2:3-diketogluconic acid which is a more potent reductant than ascorbate, and which therefore decreases further the trend for inactivating free −SH groups. The overall scheme can be schematically expressed thus

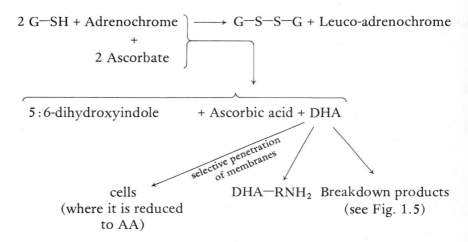

2.3. Involvement of the ascorbic system in enzymatic activities

2.3.1. General

When ascorbic acid is added to a number of enzymatic processes associated with hydroxylations, such as NADH$_2$/NAD redox interactions, significant catalysis is observed. In the past there has been a tendency to view such activities primarily in terms of oxidation/reductions involving the components of the ascorbic system. However, recent experimental observations indicate that in a number of reactions the effect may be interpreted not in terms of direct redox activities, but rather in terms of the effect of ascorbate on enzymatic *aggregation/disaggregation* as well as in contribution to *biosynthesis of enzyme components*, in particular to that of incorporation of iron into haem.

In this section we shall be concerned first with the problem of ascorbate catalytic activities when associated with a number of redox enzyme systems, such as those containing $NADH_2/NAD$, with the principles governing such reactions, and with the link between redox activity and hydroxylation activity. It is not my intention to provide

Table 2.2. Standard electrode potentials (for *reduction*) of some oxidation-reductions of biological importance

Redox System	$E_0'(\text{pH } 7.0)$
$\frac{1}{2}O_2 + 2H^+ + 2e \rightarrow H_2O$	+0.816
$Fe^{3+} + e \rightarrow Fe^{++}$	+0.771
$AFR + e \rightarrow AA$	+0.34
$\frac{1}{2}O_2 + H_2O + 2e \rightarrow H_2O_2$	+0.30
$Cu^{++} \rightarrow Cu$	+0.345
Cytochrome a $Fe^{3+} + e \rightarrow$ cytochrome a Fe^{2+}	+0.29
Cytochrome c $Fe^{3+} + e \rightarrow$ cytochrome c Fe^{2+}	+0.25
2:6-Dichlorophenolindophenol (ox) + $2H^+$ + 2e → → 2:6-Dichlorophenolindophenol (red)	+0.22
Cytochrome c_1 $Fe^{3+} + e \rightarrow$ cytochrome c_1 Fe^{2+}	+0.22
Cytochrome b_2 $Fe^{3+} + e \rightarrow$ cytochrome b_2 Fe^{2+}	+0.12 (pH 7.4)
Ubiquinone + $2H^+$ + 2e → dihydroubiquinone	+0.10
Cytochrome b_5 $Fe^{3+} + e \rightarrow$ cytochrome b_5 Fe^{2+}	+0.03
Cytochrome b $Fe^{3+} + e \rightarrow$ cytochrome b Fe^{2+}	+0.08
Dehydroascorbate + $2H^+$ + 2e → ascorbate	+0.058
$FAD + 2H \rightarrow FADH + H$	−0.05
Glutathione (ox) → glutathione (red)	−0.33
$NAD^+ \rightarrow NADH$	−0.33
$H^+ \rightarrow \frac{1}{2}H_2$	−0.42

a résumé of the research carried out in this field,* but to develop a pattern which implicates the ascorbic free radical in hydroxylation activity.

Elucidation of the mechanism of catalytic redox activities is assisted by knowledge of the standard redox potentials of the systems involved. To simplify matters, several standard redox potentials (for reduction) have been assembled in the above table (Table 2.2).

---

* For a comprehensive review of ascorbate activity in hydroxylations see Barnes and Kodicek, 1972.

2.3.2. Enzymatic catalysis of redox reactions involving the ascorbic system

One major activity of the ascorbic system is that of participation in hydroxylation* reactions—as distinct from its oxidation-reduction activity—e.g. the hydroxylation of the lysine and proline constituents of collagen. Considerable work has been carried out in this field; it will not be covered here, since adequate résumés are available in the literature (e.g. Barnes and Kodicek, 1972; Udenfriend *et al.*, 1954). Here we shall be concerned with mechanisms and energetics at the molecular level at which the ascorbate system participates in biochemical reactions. In hydroxylation reactions these can conveniently be assigned to two major factors, namely electron transfer and energy transfer which often proceed via the ascorbic free radical. The extraordinary ability of AFR to offset many reactions—to an extent far greater than that displayed by the two other constituents of the ascorbate system, AA and DHA—can be ascribed primarily to participation in one-electron transfer reactions to which the

$$Fe^{++} \; \underset{+e}{\overset{-e}{\rightleftharpoons}} \; Fe^{+++} \quad and \quad Cu^{+} \; \underset{+e}{\overset{-e}{\rightleftharpoons}} \; Cu^{++}$$

systems of the active enzyme systems are restricted. Apart from energy of activation limitations, the process

$$AA \; \underset{+2e}{\overset{-2e}{\rightleftharpoons}} \; DHA$$

required a three-body collision to collate a 2e transfer with two one-electron transfers, which compares with a two-body collision in one-electron transfers, thus making it far less likely to occur.

2.3.2.1. *Rate of reaction and range of action*

Theoretical considerations and experimental evidence lead to the conclusion that the AFR is capable of a much greater *rate* of activity

---

* Ascorbate participation in biochemical reactions sometimes exerts effects which cannot be ascribed to *direct* involvement in hydroxylations, but rather to indirect effects such as adverse effects on competing transaminase activities and participation in *de novo* synthesis of the *enzymes* involved in hydroxylation. These will be noted separately.

as well as a greater *range* of redox activity in respect of both oxidations and reductions. This is seen particularly clearly when it is *freshly formed*. See also section 2.2.3.

Rate: Because the AFR possesses a higher energy level (as a result of the unpaired electron) the energy of activation required—as compared to the two other entities of the system—is bound to be smaller. Hence, according to the equation

$$k = PZe^{-A/RT} \qquad\qquad (2.10)$$

(where k is the velocity constant, P is the probability factor, Z is the number of collisions per second, A is the energy of activation, and R and T are the gas constant and the absolute temperature respectively), the greater the concentration of AFR and the higher the excited state energy with which it is loaded, the greater is the rate.

The standard redox potential for the system AFR/AA is more positive than that of DHA/AA (~0.34 as compared with 0.058). The possession by AFR of the higher reduction emf value confers upon it a greater reducing range ability than that of the AA/DHA only system.

2.3.2.2. *Steady-state concentration of AFR and its oxidation-reducing potency*

Certain ascorbate-utilizing systems, such as peroxidase and ascorbic acid oxidase, are able to produce steady states in which the free radical is present in much larger concentrations than in those attained either under thermodynamic equilibrium conditions (on mixing of AA and DHA) or under those steady-state conditions produced by non-enzymatic processes. Such activities extend considerably the oxidation/reduction range of the ascorbic system. See also section 2.2.3.

Let us now consider the experimental evidence which supports the above pattern.

Activation of NADH oxidase by an oxidation product of ascorbate: Kern and Racker (1954) showed that NADH-oxidase activity in catalysing the oxidation of reduced NADH was stimulated by addition of ascorbic acid and even more stimulated by subsequent addition of ascorbic acid oxidase.

Kersten *et al.* (1958) used an enzyme system isolated from suprarenal microsomes for oxidation of NADH in presence of ascorbic acid and O_2. Neither DHA nor reduced glutathione could

replace ascorbic acid. They considered that AFR acts as an inter-
mediary electron acceptor in the system. Nason *et al.* (1954) also
concluded that the single-electron acceptor—which they tentatively
suggested was the ascorbic free radical—could not be formed non-
enzymatically by reduction of DHA, by reduced glutathione or
cysteine.

Iyanagi and Yamazaki (1969), on the basis of their own experimental results, suggested a possible participation of the ascorbate
free radical in microsome-catalysed oxidation of NADH.

Schneider and Staudinger (1965) examined the reduction of an
"oxidation product" of ascorbic acid with $NADH_2$ serving as
electron donor using animal microsome enzymes. They found that in
presence of the enzyme and $NADH_2$, ascorbic acid remained in the
fully reduced state even when ascorbic oxidase was added; they
concluded that in this case only the ascorbic free radical—but not
DHA—acts as electron acceptor. Their conclusion can be schematically expressed as

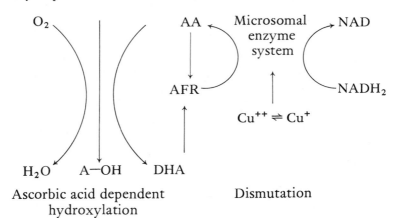

Ascorbic acid dependent   Dismutation
      hydroxylation

Reaction of AFR with cytochrome c: It can be predicted from
standard emf values and the necessary three-body collision that *AA*
would reduce cytochrome *c* non-enzymatically very slowly. However, the addition of ascorbic acid oxidase catalyses this reaction
considerably; this and the accompanying development of the ESR
spectrum of the ascorbic free radical (Yamazaki and Piette, 1961)
support the concept that the formation of AFR catalyses the
reaction effectively. The process was formulated as

$$Cyt.c^{+++} + AFR \xrightarrow{\ \ k\ \ } Cyt.c^{++} + DHA + H^+ \qquad (2.11)$$

The ratio of the enzymatic rate constant (k) to the non-enzymatic rate constant (k'), i.e. {k/k'}, was found to change from 5×10^4 (at pH 4) to 1.1×10^3 (at pH 7).

AFR can dismute into AA and DHA as well as act as an oxidant or as a reductant; in the former case it is reduced to AA, in the latter it is oxidized to DHA. In this overall process AFR acts as a reductant. The catalytic effect of ascorbic acid oxidase in activating the reduction of cytochrome c, and the co-existent dismutation of AFR can be schematically expressed as

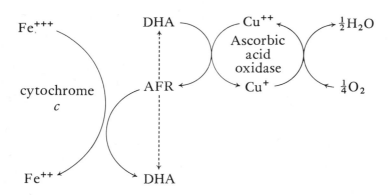

The rate constant of cytochrome c reduction by the ascorbic free radical has been computed as 4.0×10^{-4} M^{-1} sec^{-1} by Ohnishi et al. (1969).

Formation of AFR by peroxidase and by ascorbic acid oxidase: Yamazaki et al. (1959) compared the peroxidatic formation of the ascorbic free radical enzymatically and non-enzymatically at pH 4.8. The enzymatic reaction was found to be much faster than the non-enzymatic process. AFR concentrations of over 1×10^{-6} were noted. Such values are more than a thousand times greater than the equilibrium concentrations of 10^{-9} which Foerster et al. (1965) obtained on mixing of AA and DHA.

Yamazaki and Piette (1961) found that the steady state AFR concentrations formed by ascorbic acid oxidase were higher than those formed by peroxidase. They also concluded that the main pathway in both ascorbic acid oxidase and the peroxidase reactions was via the ascorbic free radical.

Reduction of cytochrome b_5. Krisch and Staudinger (1959) concluded that cytochrome b_5 is reduced by AA. Also, Hara and Minakama (1968) have suggested that AFR participates in the reduction of cytochrome b_5.

2.3.2.3. *Enzymatic hydroxylation activity of AA/AFR*

General. In line with the above observations, computations and formulations the involvement of AFR and AA *in hydroxylation reactions* is generally accepted as

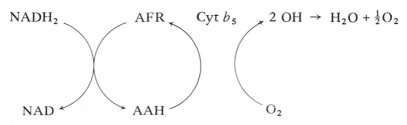

See also Mapson (1967; p. 389).

2.3.2.4. *Hydroxylation of dopamine to noradrenaline*

Dopamine can be hydroxylated—using β-dopamine hydroxylase—to noradrenaline (Levin and Kaufmann, 1961). Here also the hydroxylation is likely to proceed via AFR rather than via the AA/DHA system, as the enzyme undergoes a change of $Cu^+ \underset{+e}{\overset{-e}{\rightleftharpoons}} Cu^{++}$; indeed, Blumberg *et al.* (1965) have demonstrated that a complete incubation medium shows a small AFR signal. Blumberg *et al.* (1965) proposed a mechanism in which AFR—as the primary product of enzyme action—reacts with dopamine to produce a dopamine free radical which in turn reacts with an oxygen-complexed form of the enzyme to result in noradrenaline.

2.3.2.5. *Hydroxylation of tryptophan to form serotonin*

Ascorbate (D- or L-, or isoascorbate or DHA) has been found necessary for the first stage of formation of serotonin from tryptophan, thus

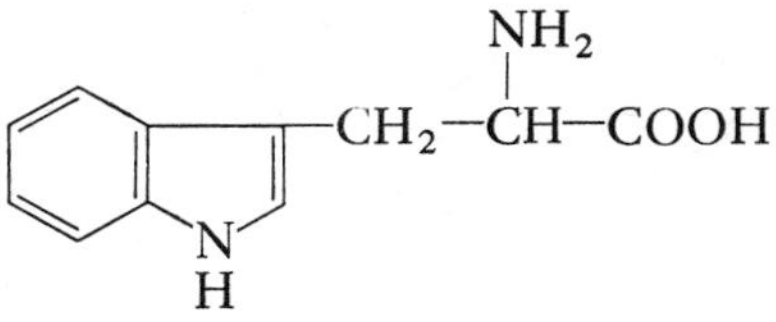

$$NH_2$$
$$CH_2-CH-COOH$$

Tryptophan

Tryptophan 5-hydroxylase
Requires L- or D-ascorbate
or DHA or isoascorbate (Cooper, 1961)

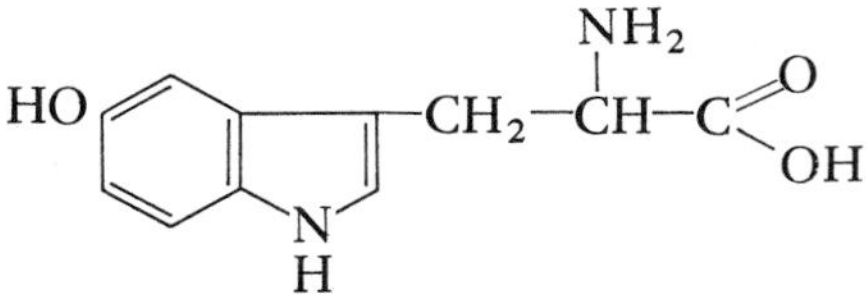

$$NH_2$$
$$HO \quad CH_2-CH-C{<}^O_{OH}$$

5-Hydroxytryptophan

5'HTP-decarboxylase

5-Hydroxytryptamine (Serotonin)

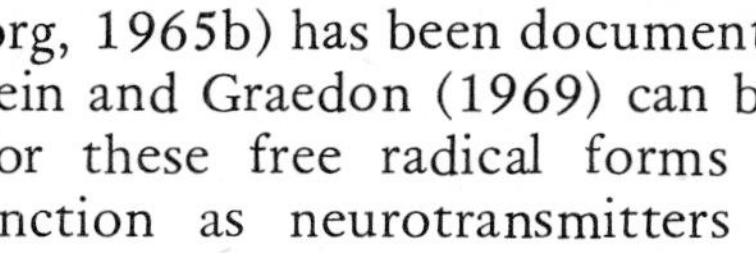

$$CH_2-CH_2-NH_2$$

The existence of free radicals of noradrenaline (Borg, 1965a) and of serotonin (Borg, 1965b) has been documented. The findings of Polis, Wyet, Goldstein and Graedon (1969) can be interpreted as supporting a role for these free radical forms when noradrenaline and serotonin function as neurotransmitters in the central nervous system.

2.3.2.6. *Hydroxylation of p-hydroxyphenylpyruvate (p-HPP) to form Homogentisate (HGA)*

Ascorbate is involved in tyrosine metabolism in the liver by participating in the conversion of p-hydroxyphenylpyruvate to

homogentisate, thus

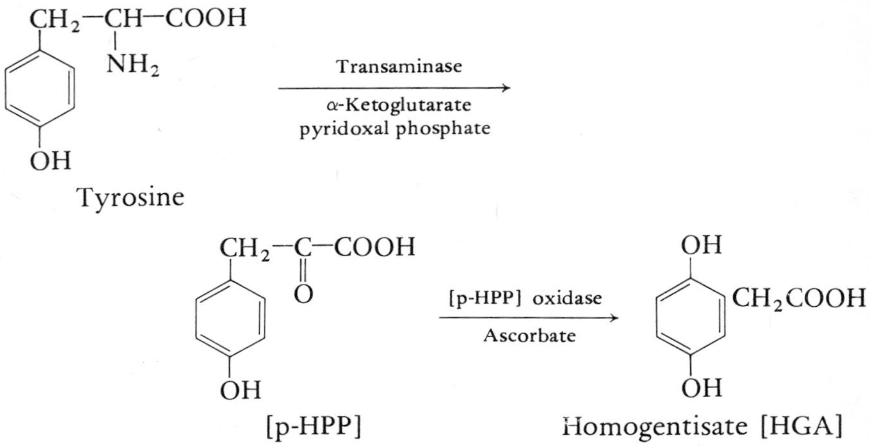

CH$_2$—CH—COOH
         |
         NH$_2$

Transaminase
————————————————————→
α-Ketoglutarate
pyridoxal phosphate

(phenol ring structure with OH)

Tyrosine

CH$_2$—C—COOH
           ‖
           O

[p-HPP] oxidase
————————————————→
Ascorbate

OH

CH$_2$COOH

OH

[p-HPP]   Homogentisate [HGA]

So far no investigations reporting the participation of ascorbic free radicals in this transformation appear to have been reported in the literature; but in view of the extensive intervention of ascorbic free radicals in hydroxylations it may well be that they also participate in this particular reaction.

2.3.3. Inhibitory effect of ascorbate on some enzyme processes

Ascorbate has been shown to exert an adverse effect on trans-amination enzyme activities and on the enzymatic decomposition of H$_2$O$_2$ by catalase:

Transamination: Srivastava and Sirohi (1969) concluded that ascorbate reduces the activity of the three transamination enzymes of glutamate-glyoxalate, glutamate-oxaloacetate, and alanine-glyoxalate.

The mechanism of this unusual activity has as yet not been elucidated energetically or at the molecular level.

Decomposition of H$_2$O$_2$: Ascorbate was found to inhibit the activity of catalase in decomposing hydrogen peroxide to water and oxygen at concentrations as low as 2×10^{-6} (Orr, 1966, 1967, 1970). Two mechanisms have been proposed; one involves a complex between H$_2$O$_2$ and the haem species of catalase, the other involves the ascorbate free radical.

Lactic acid production and oxygen uptake: High concentrations of ascorbic acid, in media in which polynuclear leucocytes (of the guinea pig) were suspended, resulted in decreased lactic acid production and increased oxygen uptake by the cells (Elliott and Smith, 1966). Parallel effects were noted on addition of ascorbate to tissue culture media of chick bone cells (Ramp and Thornton, 1968).

2.4. Effect of lowering of the interfacial tension

In order to appreciate the influence that the AA/DHA system can exert on biological equilibria by virtue of its ability to lower the interfacial tension, it is necessary to consider—albeit very briefly— how changes in interfacial tension can affect conformations and associations of biopolymers which depend on adherence and de-adherence of hydrophobic groups.

2.4.1. Interfacial tension and adherence of hydrophobic groups

Hydrophobic groups tend to adhere less strongly as the interfacial tension is lowered, and vice versa. Hence, lowering of the interfacial tension adversely affects biological conformations which rely on contributions from hydrophobic adherence. These include but-tressing of the helix in coil $\rightleftharpoons$ helix equilibria, and association of protein subunits, such as those involved in haemoglobin and in numerous enzyme systems. For example, the presence of 4M urea— which lowers the surface tension by $c.$ 9 dynes (Lewin, 1974a)—causes haemoglobin to dissociate into its 2α and 2β-subunits.

A simplified equation has been developed to relate the loss of water-surface free energy (L)—which is the driving force arising from the tendency to water extrusion—and the contact area, a, of the hydrophobic groups involved and the surface tension, γ (Lewin, 1974a). Thus,

$$L = \{3 \times 10^{-3}\gamma a\} \text{ kcal per mole/mole hydrophobic groups' adherences}$$
$$(2.12)$$

2.4.2. Adherence and de-adherence of hydrophobic groups in helix $\rightleftharpoons$ coil transformations, and in association/dissociation of protein subunits

Coil $\rightleftharpoons$ *helix transitions:* The polypeptide equilibrium

Hydrated random coils $\rightleftharpoons$ α-helix + water should tend towards the left-hand side in absence of supporting contributions from hydrophobic adherences (for discussions and references, see Lewin, 1974a). This is so because the association of initially hydrated H... donor and H... acceptor groups may by itself be insufficient to compensate for the decrease in entropy accompanying the formation of the helix. It is the loss of water-interfacial-tension free energy resulting from the adherence of suitably sited hydrophobic groups, as the helix is formed, which can tilt the balance.

Association of protein subunits: Adherence of hydrophobic groups on exposed surfaces of protein subunits enables the formation of an entity composed of these units. One case can be schematically represented as follows:

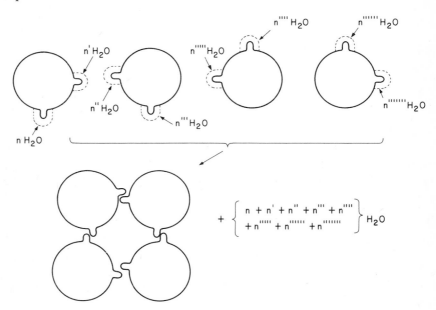

Fig. 2.2. Schematic representation of the association of four identical subunits.

The structural orientations and sitings of the hydrophobic groups must be such that the hydrophobic adherences associated with the interaction must enable only the particular association to be formed. The driving force is provided by the increase in entropy resulting from diversion of the water molecules from their highly organized state (when adjacent to the hydrophobic groups) into a less organized state in bulk water. (For details see Lewin, 1974a.) A parallel pattern to this can be used to illustrate the de-adhering effect of 4 M urea—which lowers the interfacial tension by 9 dynes/cm, a value sufficient to cause the haemoglobin to dissociate to its subunits. A similar concept can be applied to the dissociation of glutamic dehydrogenase which in 6 M urea dissociates from a multimer into a large number of monomeric subunits.

2.4.3. The potential of the AA/DHA system in respect of interfacial tension effects on adherence/de-adherence of hydrophobic groups

The force holding hydrophobic groups in contact depends on the respective magnitudes of both contact area and interfacial tension (see equation 2.12). For a given hydrophobic contact area, the value of the interfacial tension can be continuously altered from a state in which the value of L is more than sufficient to buttress a particular biopolymer conformation or association to a lower value, as a result of which the particular conformation will be disbanded by the thermal onslaught of water. Such fine control is not paralleled in other major binding forces such as H... bonding or ionic linkages. Further, the energy of hydrophobic adherence (and its control by interfacial tension) ranges from as high as several k calories to as little as 0.1 k calories, thus extending over the range of H... bonding to that of thermal-kinetic-energy (see Lewin, 1975a).

The ascorbic/dehydroascorbate system possesses a versatility even more sophisticated than other "detergent" systems which are capable of lowering the surface tension because the oxidation of AA to DHA results in increased ability to lower the interfacial tension without change of concentration. This confers increased versatility because oxidation energy can thereby be linked with hydrophobic energies and correspondingly with interfacial tension variations.

2.4.4. Dissolution of fats and cholesterol

The mild "detergent" action of the ascorbic/dehydroascorbic system enables some dissolution of fats and of cholesterol, and of cholesterol/phospholipid/Ca complexes.

Simple laboratory experiments I have carried out, using 10^{-1} or 10^{-2} M Na ascorbate show some dissolution of cholesterol and of fats. Also, a mixture of cholesterol, phospholipids and calcium salts which readily forms precipitates in test-tube experiments can be seen to display increased dissolution on introduction of increasing quantities of ascorbate. Comparisons using Na ascorbate solutions in 0.8% NaCl (to give an ionic strength which affords some protection to the ascorbate from deactivation, as well as to simulate NaCl plasma-like concentrations) display increased dissolution of the above precipitates as compared with dissolution under otherwise identical conditions in 0.8% NaCl solutions only (S. Lewin, unpublished observations); applicability of this activity to physiological conditions will be considered in Chapter 4.

2.4.5. Increased membrane permeability

It was concluded by several investigators (e.g. Martin, 1961; Hughes and Maton, 1968) that dehydroascorbic penetrates lipid membranes—such as those of erythrocytes—very much more than does ascorbate. The phenomenon has been attributed to the dehydroascorbic entity possessing a more lipid-like character than ascorbate. However, another way of viewing this phenomenon is to say that because dehydroascorbic possesses a much greater power to reduce the interfacial tension, it can correspondingly increase membrane permeability. The implications of the respective formulations are not the same:

(i) An increased lipid-like character would help the DHA to enter the membrane from the aqueous bulk, but having penetrated the membrane the DHA should prefer to stay in it because of the lipid character of the two. Hence, transfer of DHA from the plasma into the inside of the cell would not be promoted, unless the contents of the cell were themselves more lipid-like than the plasma.

(ii) According to previous explanations any *ascorbate* present with dehydroascorbic, outside the lipid membrane, need not penetrate the membrane any faster than when dehydroascorbic is absent. According to the view expressed here, the increased membrane permeability on contact with DHA should assist ascorbate penetration. Thus, in a solution containing a mixture of ascorbate and dehydroascorbic the permeability to AA should be higher than that when ascorbate alone is present.

Chapter 3

Vitamin C determination: Scope and limitations of interpretation

3.1. Sources of error

Much work has been carried out on the development of techniques suitable for the determination of ascorbate and its products in various tissues and other media. This research has been complicated by the need to eliminate interference with the assay procedures by other substances. The experimental techniques that have been developed can conveniently be divided into chemical methods, radioactive tracer determinations, enzymatic techniques, column, paper and thin layer separation techniques, and gas chromatography.* It is not the purpose of this chapter to review the literature, but to discuss briefly the problems that arise in assaying ascorbic acid and to point out sources of error which have not been sufficiently well appreciated; in particular, this chapter gives details of my investigations showing that cyclic AMP phosphodiesterase can hydrolyse the lactose structure of the vitamin, and then suggests procedures by which errors in assay can be avoided. The existence of these errors and failure to account for hydrolysis of ascorbic acid can cause erroneous interpretations in evaluating the relative importance of various biosynthetic and catabolic paths and thus in establishing the requirements of biological species for the vitamin.

Misconceptions may arise at the following stages:
  (a) Erroneous assumptions in respect of the values of intake and excretion of ascorbate and its products.
  (b) Errors in the experimental assay.
  (c) Errors in interpretation concerning the biosynthesis and metabolism of vitamin C.

---

* References to these techniques are given in Bibliography III.

3.1.1. Erroneous assumptions concerning the magnitude of intake of vitamin C

Vitamin C can be administered orally, intravenously or intraperitoneally.

3.1.1.1. *Oral intake**

Orally, vitamin C is administered in tablets or in solution. Either method can involve a significant error in the assumption that the dose taken does indeed contain the presumed quantity of the vitamin.

Tablets. In my experience some effervescent tablets of ascorbate manufactured by two well-known firms showed brown discoloration within a year or two of being kept at room temperature; but the phenomenon was far less pronounced when they were kept in the refrigerator at *c.* 4°C. Using spectrophotometry and optical rotation as criteria, I have noted in some of the tablets deactivation of as much as 50% to 80% of the original content of ascorbate over six months to a year. When bottles containing the tablets were kept in a desiccator at room temperature, the contents were much more stable than when no attempt was made at desiccation. When the desiccator containing the bottles of tablets was kept in the refrigerator and covered with dark paper the deterioration was of the order of 0.5% to 2% within a year. When the bottles were first flushed with nitrogen free from oxygen, then kept under nitrogen in a desiccator in a refrigerator at 4°C for two years, the deterioration was less than 1%. The deteriorating effect can be attributed to the hygroscopic activity of the tablets enabling cooperative participation of light, oxygen and water in the deactivation of the vitamin (see also Chapter 1). As ideal preserving conditions are often not enforced in the case of bottles containing vitamin C preparations, it is not surprising to find some degradation. In contrast tablets or powder of ascorbic *acid*—in the absence of bicarbonate—which have been kept in air in the dark at the temperature range of 10 to 25°C mostly showed very little deterioration even after two years (less than 0.5%).

Solution. Solutions of *ascorbate* are degraded rapidly even under anaerobic conditions (see Chapter 1) unless chelating agents such as amino acids are added. Thus in experiments in which an assayed dose of ascorbate is quoted, the amount actually present could very well

---

* See also sections 7.2.1 and 7.2.2.

be significantly lower depending on the interval of time between preparation and administration, extent of exposure to light, and content of unchelated multivalent cations such as those of copper and iron.

The oral intake of ascorbate is also subject to hazards of ascorbate degradation in the duodenum where ample oxygen is still present and the pH of the solution is neutral or slightly alkaline.

Slow-release capsules are useful in that the loss while passing the duodenum should be comparatively small. However, so far no experimental data appear to be available in this connection.

3.1.1.2. *Intravenous injection (and intraperitoneal injection)*

Intravenous injection of ascorbate solution has been used in many experiments resulting in much more rapid absorption than in the case of oral intake. However, it is necessary to emphasize that even freshly prepared ascorbate solutions—in distilled water or in physiological saline, in air, in the absence of chelating agents—can deteriorate rapidly. As much as 30 to 50% deactivation may be encountered within an hour at 20° to 30°C, depending on the iron or copper content of the ascorbic source and the incidence of light (see also Morton, 1942).

Ampules of ascorbate solution cannot be relied on to contain the assayed quantities of the vitamin unless the various precautions noted above have been enforced both in the preparation and in storing of the solutions prior to injection.

3.2. Errors in interpretation of experimental data on metabolism and excretion of vitamin C and its products

3.2.1. Location and excretion

In order to appreciate the possible extent of error in interpretation of experimental data on excretion of vitamin C in relation to its metabolism and on relevant fixing of the "daily allowance" (i.e. the quantity of vitamin C to be recommended as sufficient for upkeep of health in human beings), it is essential to consider the various loci in which vitamin C can be present and the various catabolic paths to which vitamin C can be subject in humans. Figure 3.1 represents the various possibilities.

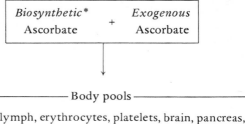

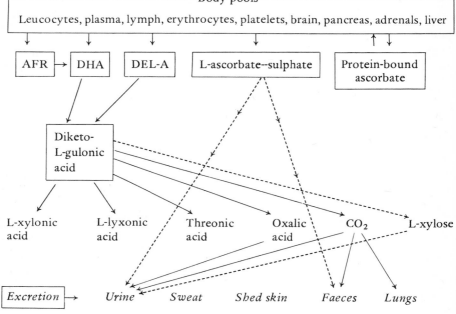

Fig. 3.1. Schematic representation of input and excretion of body ascorbate.

* See sections 5.4 and 8.2.

3.2.2. Ascorbate balance

As will be appreciated from Fig. 3.1 there are various sites in which ascorbate can exist in the body before and during its metabolism. The half-life of ascorbate associated with a particular catabolic path may well differ from those following other paths, thereby making the "average" half-life a nominal figure. (See also section 5.5.2 for discussion of the fate of ascorbate upon metabolism.) Experiments using radioactive tracers resulted in the range of values for average half-lives for humans shown in Table 3.1.

The question arising from these data is: to what extent do biochemical individuality, errors inherent in the assays themselves,

Table 3.1. Variations in half-life of ascorbate in humans

Half-life	Source
13–20 days	Hellman and Burns (1958)
16 days	Burns et al. (see Burns, 1967)
8–24 days	Baker et al. (1966)
13–30 days	Abt et al. (1963)

and erroneous assumptions in the calculations of half-life, contribute to the apparent variations seen in this range of values?

Changes in biochemical individuality must obviously contribute to the variations in computed values. Indeed, even a particular individual can display considerable variations as a result of change in diet. For example, subsequent to a control period, ingestion of 300 mg of pyridoxine hydrochloride for 30 days—although not resulting in change in the computed ascorbic acid pool size—was followed by an increased rate of ascorbate utilization from 21-22 mg per day to 62-70 mg per day as expressed in oxalate production (Baker, Sauberlich, Amos and Tollotson, 1966).

In general, computations of ascorbic pool size and of efficiency of ascorbate utilization rely on the dogma that no ascorbate whatsoever is biosynthesized in human tissues. The basic relationship adopted is thus:

Amount of ingested ascorbate =

[*ascorbate* in the various tissues]
+
[*ascorbate-products* in various tissues]
+
[*ascorbate* excreted in urine and faeces]
+
[*ascorbate-products* excreted in urine and faeces]

However, in view of the evidence marshalled in Chapters 5 and 8 this dogma is not tenable. Only one example need be quoted at this stage. The original calculations published prior to 1971 (e.g. Baker *et al.*, 1966; Baker, 1967; Burns *et al.*, 1967) accounted for only ascorbate, diketoglutonate, traces of CO_2 and oxalate presence in the urine (and faeces) and a small percentage of "unknowns". Some were based on findings that "the summation of urinary oxalate and urinary ascorbate equalled the total amount of radioactivity found in the urine, both in cumulative total and for each individual day" (Baker, Saari and Tolbert, 1966). Yet the ingested radioactive ascorbate accounted for was noted to be in the low range of 67 to 79%, for which no satisfactory explanation was available. Also the recent isolation of L-ascorbate sulphate in human urine and that of other animals indicates a source of loss of which account must be taken. The findings of Baker *et al.* (1971) are that about 3% of the body pool of ascorbate (i.e. *c.* 3% × (2.6 to 2.8 g) namely *c.* 71 mg are metabolized per day as L-ascorbate sulphate. Taken in conjunction with 20–40 mg ascorbate metabolized per day in the case of presumably healthy men with presumably as high a level of intake as 70 mg per day (the recommended dietary allowance in the U.S.A.), one is faced with a loss in the human urine of about 100 mg per day, i.e. an excess of *c.* 30 mg ascorbate per day,* which suggests an endogenous source of ascorbate. Indeed Baker *et al.* (1962) have observed that ingestion of D-glucurono-α-lactone in some volunteers resulted in the formation of ascorbic acid. The considerations in favour of the thesis that humans do produce insufficient quantities of ascorbate will be followed in Chapters 5 and 8. Here however we are concerned with the thesis that the unsatisfactory accounting for ingested ascorbate results in uncertainty as to the *degree* of validity of published computations of ascorbate metabolic paths, particularly when extrapolations are attempted from the results of isotopically labelled exogenous ascorbate.

3.3. De-lactonization of ascorbate by 3′,5′-cyclic AMP-phosphodiesterase (PDE)

3.3.1. De-lactonization of DHA and of ascorbate

It has been known for some time that the lactone structure of DHA can be hydrolytically ruptured by aldonolactonases (also known as gulono-γ-lactone hydrolases), e.g. Kagawa and Takiguchi (1961) and Kawada *et al.* (1960).† However, despite extensive search of the literature no information regarding enzymatic hydrolysis of

---

* Indeed, this value is likely to be too low an estimate because it does not include losses following delactonization of ascorbate by hydrolytic action of c-AMP-phosphodiesterase, as will be outlined later on.

† Lactonase activity can be measured by CO_2 displacement from bicarbonate in Warburg flasks (e.g. Yamada, Ishikawa and Shimazono, 1959).

L-ascorbic acid was found. The de-lactonization may be represented as

$$
\begin{array}{c}
\text{H--C} \overset{\displaystyle |}{} \overset{O}{\diagdown} \text{C}{=}O \\
\text{C}{=}\text{C} \\
\overset{|}{\text{OH}} \quad \overset{|}{\text{OH}}
\end{array}
\;+\;H_2O \;\longrightarrow\;
\begin{array}{c}
\text{H--C} \overset{\displaystyle |}{} OH \quad \overset{OH}{\underset{|}{\text{C}}}{=}O \\
\text{C}{=}\text{C} \\
\overset{|}{\text{OH}} \quad \overset{|}{\text{OH}}
\end{array}
$$

The hydrolysed form still possesses the double bond between C-2 and C-3 and the respective OH groups in C-2 and C-3 in the unionized form; it is a good reducing agent, and has $\lambda_{max} = 275$ nm and can be transformed into the lactone form by digestion in 8% HCl at 50°C (Haworth and Hirst, 1933). It must be emphasized that the de-lactonized form is *biologically inactive.*

3.3.2. De-lactonization of L-ascorbate by the hydrolytic activity of PDE

Both 3'-5':cyclic AMP and ascorbate possess ring structures formed as a result of water elimination, and each has a negatively charged oxygen atom attached to the ring. Now cyclic AMP has been shown to be hydrolysed by c-AMP-phosphodiesterase (PDE). In view of the similarity between cyclic AMP and ascorbate, I considered it feasible that the lactone ring structure of ascorbate may well be hydrolysed by PDE. A search of the literature showed that Moffat *et al.* (1972) established chromatographically that ascorbate is one of those substances which exert an inhibitory action on the hydrolysis of cyclic AMP by PDE. This finding could readily be accommodated within the conceptual framework that both ascorbate and c-AMP can be hydrolysed by PDE and that the inhibiting trend by ascorbate on the hydrolysis of c-AMP by PDE is due to a competition for the active sites in PDE. I therefore undertook an investigation into possible hydrolytic activity of PDE on ascorbate. Numerous experiments in the range of pH 7.5 to 8 with PDE showed that the enzyme acts on ascorbate to liberate acid. The pH statting method, employing automatic pH statting, was used. Various ascorbate and PDE concentrations were employed. The following is given in illustration: 3 ml of a mixture [containing 0.18 mg PDE (Sigma),* 0.05 M NaCl, 0.0001 M Mg^{++} and 0.0001 M Na ascorbate, initially rapidly

---

* E.C.3.1.4.1.7.

adjusted to pH 8.0 at 30°C] was kept anaerobic by bubbling in N_2 (free from O_2 and CO_2). Exposure to light during preparation and experimental run was avoided as far as possible. 3×10^{-3} N NaOH was used as titrant. A short incubation period was usually observed; it was followed by automatic titration with NaOH to keep the pH constant.*

It was found necessary to use *freshly prepared* stock PDE† solution and stock Na ascorbate in order to obtain end-points which were within the region of equivalence. The "best" results gave end-points between 80 and 90% of the equivalent of ascorbate (assuming that each ascorbate molecule was delactonized) and were obtained when freshly prepared stock ascorbate solutions had $\epsilon_{max\ 265.5} \geqslant 20,000$ and when simultaneous spectrophotometric checks at 265.5 nm at 30°C under anaerobic conditions showed that the optical density value remained constant during the experimental period. Figure 3.2 illustrates two of the results obtained. Increasing age of the stock solutions, and in particular exposure to light, gave rise to erratic results which sometimes could be foreseen as a simultaneous spectrophotometric check showed a steady fall-off in the optical absorbance.

This method suffers from the prohibition on the use of chelating agents which stabilize ascorbate against degradation, which is necessary because these agents will also remove the free ionic species of Mg^{++}, Mn^{++}, Co^{++} and Zn^{++} without which PDE becomes inactive. The precautions required in the execution of the method are such that its general use for assaying ascorbate may be considered impractical. Currently, its physiological significance lies in its ability to demonstrate the breakdown of ascorbate, by PDE, to an acid which, in view of the exclusion of aerobic conditions (and the steadiness of the optical density), is likely to be the result of

---

* Thanks are due to various helpers (e.g. R. Stoker, G. Stubbs and P. Marshall) for checks and rechecks of the pH statting period.

† PDEs from other sources gave somewhat different results. Overall, the deviations could be due to the presence of different proportions of the two different forms of PDE and the protein activator which would be deactivated at different rates. It is relevant to note that Brooker *et al.* (1968) recorded that PDE from rat brain has two Km values, one of *c.* 10^{-4} M, the other *c.* 10^{-6} M; Cheung (1970) and Cheung and Patrick (1970) reported the involvement of a protein activator in PDE activity. Tisdale (1975) reported that PDE from Walker's carcinoma behaves kinetically as possessing a low affinity activity (Km 82.5 μM) and a high affinity activity (Km 2.3 μM), and that both ascorbate and DHA are reversible inhibitors of the enzyme with inhibitors' constants comparable to theophylline. Buck and Zadunaisky (1975) reported that ascorbate inhibits PDE from subcellular homogenates of corneal epithelium and other tissues; 5 mM and 20 mM ascorbate resulted in 16% and 46% inhibitions respectively in comparison with a 56% inhibition by 5 mM theophylline.

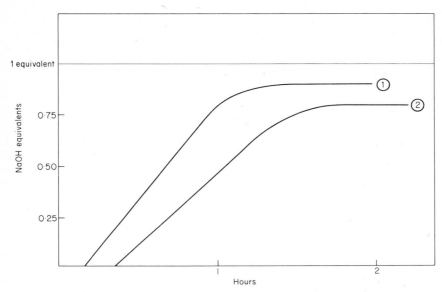

Fig. 3.2. pH statting of the reaction of ascorbate with PDE. 30°C. Anaerobic conditions. 3 ml of a solution containing 0.18 mg PDE (*freshly* prepared; Sigma), 5×10^{-2} M NaCl, 10^{-4} M MgCl$_2$, and 10^{-4} M ascorbate (*freshly* prepared) were pH stated with 3×10^{-3} N NaOH.

delactonization. It is hoped that as a result of current researches, which include thin layer chromatography and radioactive tracer techniques, additional supporting evidence will become available.

3.4. Resultant issues

The hydrolysis of the lactone structure of ascorbate by PDE raises numerous experimental problems and theoretical questions, some of which are as follows:

1. What are the subsequent metabolic/physiological activities of the delactonized ascorbate (DEL-A)?

2. What is the effect on the calculations of the body metabolic ascorbate pool?

3. To what extent is DEL-A re-lactonized to AA in different tissues?

4. To what extent does the competition between ascorbate and cyclic nucleotides for the active sites of PDE involve control of endocrinal and "second" messenger activities of c-AMP and c-GMP?

5. To what extent does mega intake of AA compensate—or

over-compensate—for the "loss" of the lactone as a result of hydrolysis by PDE?

These and other aspects will be discussed in subsequent chapters as appropriate. However, it cannot be overemphasized at this stage that vitamin C assays on biological materials in the past may have been significantly in error as a result of non-inclusion of DEL-A in the calculations.

3.5. The reaction of ascorbate with α,α-diphenyl-β-picrylhydrazyl (DPPH˙)

Blois (1958) showed that ascorbate reacts with the free radical DPPH˙ in the ratio of one ascorbate to two DPPH˙, and that the reaction can be conveniently followed at 517 mμ in acetate buffers in the pH region of 5.0 to 6.5 [see section 1.3.5.3].

Ascorbate is biologically active whereas DEL-A is not (Haworth and Hirst, 1933). Much of the biological potential of ascorbate is due to its ability to form AFR and to inhibit PDE activity. It follows that DEL-A may not possess the potential of vitamin activity because it is not able to carry out these functions. If this is the case, DEL-A would not react as readily—or in the same way—as ascorbate does with DPPH˙. Preliminary experiments I have carried out suggest that this is the case, and it is hoped that work in progress will enable the development of an experimental procedure leading to a clear-cut assay for ascorbate.

It is hoped that in future a combination of a suitable procedure of PDE assay of ascorbate by pH statting, and a spectrophotometric assay of the ascorbate reaction with DPPH˙, contrasted with an overall assay of {DEL-A + ascorbate} using other methods such as titration with 2:6 dichlorophenolindophenol will enable differential assays of AA and DEL-A.

Part II

Biological effects

Chapter 4

Biological activity and potential

4.1. *Modus operandi* of ascorbate

Ascorbate can exercise significant influence on biological activities in various ways:

Directly, that is via its characteristic physicochemical properties of ionized state, oxidation/reduction, its capacity to lower interfacial tension, and H... bonding participation.

Indirectly, by

(i) Influencing the concentration levels of the cyclic nucleotides c-AMP and c-GMP.

(ii) Affecting the *level of enzymatic activity*.

(iii) Involvement in *hormone production*, such as that of adrenaline, noradrenaline and serotonin.

(iv) Influencing *enzyme biosynthesis*. The findings that ascorbate is present in *nuclei* of calf-thymus and liver (Stern and Timonen, 1954) and that ascorbate enhances RNA biosynthesis in wheat *nuclei* (Price, 1966) raise the possibility of an involvement in activities impinging on biosynthesis at the genetic level.

(v) *Detoxicating activity* of endogenous toxic and exogenous toxic substances. The former case can be illustrated by the reducing action of ascorbate on toxic substances such as adrenochrome* (which interferes with many enzymatic reactions) and by elimination of compounds which interfere with deactivation of neurotransmitters, such as the action of acetylcholine esterase on acetylcholine. The latter case is exemplified by the increased resistance by rats to lethal doses of barbiturates, when given vitamin C (Einhauser, 1939) and similarly by humans to the toxic effects of Pb^{++} (e.g. Marin, 1941) and Hg^{++} (Marchmont-Robinson, 1941).

---

* See sections 1.3.5.5 and 2.2.5.

(vi) *Anti-histamine activity.* This is highly useful in those biochemical stress conditions in which excessive quantitites of
histamine are formed (e.g. Businco, 1949). See also section
1.3.4.2 and section 4.4.6.

Combined activities in tissue repair, e.g. in the formation of
collagen required for healing damaged tissues.

4.2. Ascorbate content as indication of potential activities

4.2.1. Significance of different tissue concentrations

Several body tissues contain higher concentrations of ascorbate
than plasma. Such a situation must involve active transport (i.e.
against the concentration gradient). Mechanisms by which such
transfers can take place will be considered in Chapter 6. Here we
shall be concerned with the tissue content and the *uses* to which
ascorbate can be put.

4.2.2. Variation in ascorbate content of the tissues

The experimentally determined values for a given tissue can vary
significantly with the individual's age, with different individuals of
the same age and with the investigation—since strict comparisons of
individuals are not possible in post-mortems with different time
intervals between death and the post-mortem—and with different
procedures adopted by different investigators. The determined values
of ascorbate content in the adrenals can be used in illustration. (All
data quoted here have been adjusted, for the sake of comparison, to
mg ascorbate per kilo of wet tissue.) Roston (1962) gives the highest
average value of 4000 to 5000; Yavorsky *et al.*'s (1934) highest value
is 1300; while Giroud's (1938) highest value is for fetuses, 1820, and
for newborn infants, 700; Lloyd and Sinclair (1953) give 970 to
1600.

It is apposite to point out one source of error which must be
difficult to overcome, namely that of the time required for the
preparation of the various extracts from the tissues. The longer the
period during which the extract is in contact with macerated tissue,
the greater is the amount of ascorbate likely to be lost as a result of
oxidation, double-bond elimination or hydrolytic rupture of the ring.
This can readily be checked by plotting the rate of decrease in
optical density (in physiological pH range) at 265.5 nm of the

extracted liquid from which all the macerated material has been removed or subsequent to the addition of a known quantity of ascorbate. Even at 5°C as much as 10% can be lost within the first quarter of an hour, unless special precautions are taken to use very dim lighting and to eliminate free multivalent cations and oxygen.

Another source of error is concerned with the adrenals themselves. When excised adrenals are kept unmacerated even for a short time, the constituent adrenaline is rapidly oxidized to adrenochrome; the latter oxidizes ascorbate to dehydroascorbic (see sections 1.3.5.5 and 2.2.5).

Bearing in mind the different extents of probability of deactivation of tissue ascorbate, the order of the level of ascorbate content in various tissues can nevertheless be presented as

$$\text{Adrenals} > \begin{cases} \text{Leucocytes,} \\ \text{Pituitary} \end{cases} > \text{Brain} > \begin{cases} \text{Eye-lens,} \\ \text{Pancreas} \end{cases} >$$

$$\begin{cases} \text{Kidney,} \\ \text{Liver,} \\ \text{Spleen} \end{cases} > \text{Heart-muscle} > \text{Plasma}$$

Table 4.1 gives the *averaged* values of ascorbate content of various tissues. For further details, such as method of assay, any recorded vitamin C intake, and variations in individual values, the various reviews and original references should be consulted.

4.2.3. Tissue content and function

The lowest recorded ascorbate content of tissue is that of plasma. Active transport must therefore enforce removal of ascorbate from blood and lymph to tissues containing higher ascorbate concentrations. Several factors may be responsible for high content of ascorbate:

(i) Convenience of site for storage,
(ii) active utilization site for biochemical interactions, and
(iii) transport activity itself.

It is now apposite to consider the significance of the ascorbate content of several of the tissues in these terms.

Table 4.1. Ascorbate content (mg/kg wet weight) of human tissue (averaged values from the references)

Tissue	Fetuses	Newly born	Children	Adults	Old people	Reference
Adrenals			1190			Bessey and King (1933)
	1820	700	500	400	100	Giroud (1938)
		780	760			Ingalls (1939)
		581	540	393	230	Yavorsky et al. (1934)
		(4000 → 5000, unspecified age)				Roston (1962)
Leucocytes		(250 → 350, unspecified age)				Masek and Hruba (1964)
		(250 → 350, unspecified age)				Lowry et al. (1946)
Brain		460	310		110	Yavorsky et al. (1934)

(For contents of cerebral cortex and cerebellar cortex see section 4.6)

Tissue	Newly born / Children / Adults	Reference
Pituitary	889 (0-9); 950 (10-14) 770 (20-29 yrs) (yrs) (yrs) 488 (30-39 yrs) 447 (40-49 yrs) 521 (50-59 yrs) 511 (60-69 yrs) 497 (70-79 yrs) 455 (80-89 yrs)	Schaus (1957)
(Hypophysis)	750 (24 yrs, female); 650 (48 yrs, male)	Melka (1936)
Eye lens	310	Euler and Malmberg (1936)

(For extensive analysis of eye tissues see Tables 4.2 and 4.3)

Tissue	Fetuses	Newly born	Children	Adults	Old people	Reference
Pancreas		365	265	152	95	Yavorsky et al. (1934)
			300 (20 mnths)			
Thymus		304	255		46	Yavorsky et al. (1934)
Kidney		153	110	98	47	Yavorsky et al. (1934)
	350	100	70	50	30	Giroud (1938)
Liver		149	155	135	64	Yavorsky et al. (1934)
			370 (20 mnths)			Bessey and King (1933)

Table 4.1—*continued*

Tissue	Fetuses	Newly born	Children	Adults	Old people	Reference
			200	150	40	Giroud (1938)
		385				Ingalls (1939)
Spleen		155	135	127	81	Yavorsky *et al.* (1934)
Myocardium		73 (0–9 yrs) decreasing to 49 (80–89 yrs)				Schaus (1957)

4.3. Activity of ascorbate in the adrenals

4.3.1. Formation and protection of noradrenaline and adrenaline

Several hormones are formed in the adrenal medulla, e.g. noradrenaline and adrenaline; they are then transported elsewhere after passing through the cortex. These two hormones require ascorbate for formation and for protection from oxidation. These needs can be appreciated from Fig. 4.1.

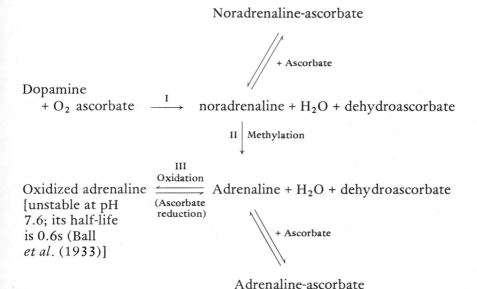

Noradrenaline-ascorbate

+ Ascorbate

Dopamine
+ O_2 ascorbate $\xrightarrow{\text{I}}$ noradrenaline + H_2O + dehydroascorbate

II | Methylation

III
Oxidation

Oxidized adrenaline $\rightleftarrows$ Adrenaline + H_2O + dehydroascorbate
[unstable at pH   (Ascorbate
7.6; its half-life   reduction)
is 0.6s (Ball   + Ascorbate
et al. (1933)]

Adrenaline-ascorbate

Fig. 4.1. Schematic representation of the ascorbate-assisted formation of adrenaline from dopamine.

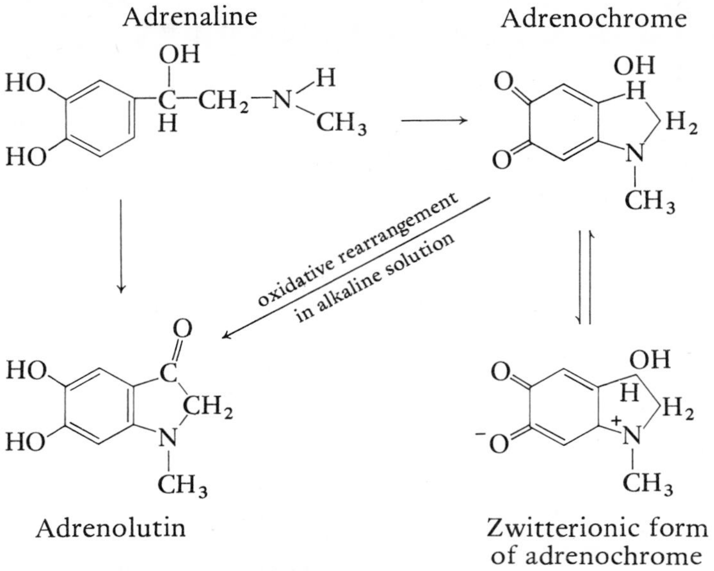

Adrenaline — Adrenochrome

Fig. 4.2. Relationship between adrenaline, adrenochrome and adrenolutin.

Adrenaline and noradrenaline, in the absence of ascorbate, are oxidized to their respective adrenochromes; the case of adrenaline is illustrated in Fig. 4.2.

4.3.2. Toxicity of oxidation products of noradrenaline and adrenaline

It must be emphasized that adrenochrome is a highly toxic substance: it can exhibit toxicity in concentrations as low as 10^{-6} to 10^{-7} M. It does this by interfering with normal enzymatic reactions. The following experimental evidence illustrates its toxicity.

Park *et al.* (1956a, b) found that at 5×10^{-4} M adrenochrome completely uncoupled oxidative phosphorylation in hamster and liver mitochondria and that glutathione prevented this uncoupling.

Krall *et al.* (1964) reported that at 5×10^{-5} M adrenochrome inhibited pyruvate oxidation and accompanying phosphorylation by 50% in brain mitochondria. This was ascribed to adrenochrome binding of the free sulphydryl groups on the enzyme.

Roston (1965) reported that the presence of the oxidized form of adrenaline resulted in accelerated disappearance of the sulphydryl group of glutathione, in the red cell.

Inchiosa and VanDenmark (1958) and Inchiosa and Freedberg (1961) found that 10^{-6} to 10^{-7} M adrenochrome inhibited ATPase activity.

Denisov (1964) noted that adrenochrome adversely affected heart muscle myosin ATPase activity.

Adrenochrome inhibits acetylcholine-esterase activity (Waelsch and Rachow, 1942). (These authors suggested that this activity could result in a positive feedback system which would disrupt the parasympathetic-sympathetic biochemical cycles. The inhibition would in turn elevate acetylcholine levels thereby raising the action of adrenaline and noradrenaline and hence adrenochrome levels thus inhibiting the esterase still further.)

Holtz and Westerman (1956) recorded that adrenochrome is a powerful inhibitor of glutamic acid decarboxylase.

4.3.3. Protection from oxidation

Complementary H... bonding between 5,6-dihydroxycatechol groups and ascorbate can protect adrenaline and noradrenaline from aerobic oxidation to their respective aminochromes (see section 1.2.8.3). Additionally, aminochromes once formed can be reduced by ascorbic acid to their respective 5,6-dihydroxy-N-methylindoles. The mechanism of reduction of adrenochrome in aqueous solution or methanol was examined by spectroscopy (Mattock, 1965) and polarography (Seelert and Schenk, 1966). Free radicals and the undisssociated form of ascorbic acid were implicated as intermediates in the reaction, on using EPR measurements. The various stages in the reduction have been outlined in sections 1.3.5.5 and 2.2.5. Hence, ascorbate/ascorbic acid, by reducing and thereby eliminating adrenochrome, removes a powerful source of toxicity and inter-ference with normal physiological activity.

4.4. White blood cells and ascorbate activity

4.4.1. Ascorbate concentration and white cell activity

The concentration of ascorbate in leucocytes is one of the highest known and is considered to be second only to that in the adrenals.

Experimentally it has been established that certain classes of antibodies are produced in leucocytes, and that that lysozomes of the phagocytes are involved in active disintegration of foreign bodies.

Recently, it has been noted that leucocytes move towards infarcted coronary sites and deposit ascorbate there (Hume *et al.*, 1972). This observation lends additional support to the concept that leucocytes are actively engaged in transporting large quantities of ascorbate to damaged tissues to an extent greater than that possible using blood or lymph in the absence of leucocytes because of the threshold limit of *c*. 1.4 to 2.4. mg ascorbate per 100 ml of plasma enforced by the kidneys. Several definite or likely functions of leucocytes involving ascorbate will now be discussed, including protein synthesis, phagocytosis, and formation of cyclic AMP.

4.4.2. Formation of γ-globulins

Leucocytes are involved in the production of γ-globulins—generally known as antibodies—which contain a large number of disulphide bonds, relative to the smaller number present in other proteins, whose function is to bridge the light and heavy chains. Disulphide bonds are not provided by amino acids added to the primary polypeptide chain during protein synthesis, but during the biosynthesis of proteins containing S—S links the individual chains are synthesized using cysteine in the amino acid sequence. Only subsequently are the corresponding and complementary —SH groups of the chains oxidized to generate cystine by oxidants such as DHA. Thus maintenance of ascorbate concentration at a high level in leucocytes should help attain the comparatively rapid oxidation/reduction activity that is required in the overall synthesis of γ-globulins.

Proteins in ingested food contain the sulphydryl/disulphide system mostly in the disulphide form, because of the increased probability of previous aerobic oxidation, and are thus incorporated into the body upon digestion. To attain the sulphydryl form required for use in protein biosynthesis, reduction is necessary, and this may be enhanced by availability of nascent AFR (see section 2.2.3). Further, the concentration of substances which oxidize available thiol groups—e.g. adrenochrome—is decreased (or eliminated) by ascorbate (see section 1.3.5.5).

4.4.3. Ascorbate transport by leucocytes

It has been known for some time that white blood corpuscles converge on infected and on wounded areas. However, attention has been focused on ingestion and destruction of bacteria mainly by phagocytic action, using the lysozomes, and by making available antibodies for attacking the bacterial invaders. It has also been recognized for quite some time that vitamin C is helpful in the repair of damaged tissues, particularly as it participates in the formation of collagen in the tissues being newly formed. If we now collate the various available observations, the emerging picture is that a major function of the leucocytes is to transport vitamin C to damaged tissues to assist in the biosynthesis of protein forming part of the new tissues. Since the high concentration of ascorbate in leucocytes must involve active transport (i.e. anti-concentration gradient) from the plasma, it is relevant to pose the question as to what processes can be visualized to cause the leucocytes to discharge their stored ascorbate into the damaged tissues. This aspect will be considered in Chapter 6.

4.4.4. Phagocytosis

Phagocytosis, i.e. the ingestion and destruction of bacteria by phagocytes—also termed polymorphonuclear leucocytes—has long been known to be one of the chief defence mechanisms of the body against bacterial attack.

The ability of phagocytes to carry out such activities has been shown to be associated with adequate presence of ascorbate in the white cells. That individuals with low vitamin levels display low phagocyte activity has been ascertained by various investigators (e.g. Merchant, 1950; Busing, 1942; Cottingham and Mills, 1943) using related criteria such as resistance of the leucocytes to fragility, pseudopoid formation, motility and the number of bacteria ingested per cell. The trend of the results can be appreciated from the following.

Mills (1949)—using guinea pigs over a period of four weeks—showed that increasing doses of ascorbic acid (to 0.5, 1.5 and 3.0 mg per day per guinea pig) resulted in the number of ingested bacteria per phagocyte increasing significantly with the dose. The trend can be illustrated by the following results obtained at 68°F:

Ascorbic acid (mg/pig/day)	0.5	1.5	3.0
Bacteria/cell	7.42 (±0.56)	11.90 (±0.38)	12.02 (±0.59)

Parallel results were obtained in other series of experiments carried out at 90–91°F under 60–70% relative humidities.

Nungster and May (1948) related, *inter-alia*, the vitamin C level of guinea pig serum with the phagocytic activity of the leucocytes. Their results clearly established that increased activity of the phago-cytes (accompanied by decreased fragility) accompanied increase in the vitamin C level of the corresponding serum.

4.4.5. Formation and transport of cyclic-AMP

Leucocytes are expected to contain adenyl-cyclase that can be stimulated by catecholamines to potentiate c-AMP formation [see Table 6-III in Robison, Butcher and Sutherland (1971), page 216; also Scott (1970)]. Now, ascorbate inhibits the hydrolysis of c-AMP by phosphodiesterase (see Chapter 3). It could therefore well be that one of the functions of high ascorbate concentration in the leuco-cytes is the upkeep of sufficiently high level of c-AMP and its transport to the required site.

4.4.6. Anti-histamine effect

Histamine is found stored, in the mammalian body, within tissue mast cells or basophil leucocytes; it is released by various drugs and antigens, but cyclic AMP inhibits this release (Kakiuchi and Rall, 1968a, b; Shimizu *et al.*, 1969). Indeed, Busieno (1949) concluded that ascorbic acid and nicotinamide in the guinea pig are the most potent anti-histamine substances. Histamine is also known to depress the ascorbic acid content of the adrenal cortex. Schayer (1962) recorded that histamine production is increased considerably in response to biochemical stress such as burns, infection and adminis-tration of several drugs. Also, Subramanian *et al.* (1973) concluded that one function of ascorbate is detoxification of excess of hist-amine produced in response to biochemical stress. It has also been found that β-adrenergic catecholamines exert an inhibitory effect on the antigen-induced histamine release. Lichtenstein and Margolis (1968) and Assem and Schild (1969) have shown that the above inhibitory effect of catecholamines is reduced by c-AMP. Histamine is known to influence c-AMP levels (e.g. Rall and Kakiuchi, 1966). Thus, a considerable extent of interplay of histamine and c-AMP takes place. As will be pointed out (see section 4.9.2.3) ascorbate enhances high c-AMP levels, and hence an indirect relationship between histamine and ascorbate can be presumed. It is therefore interesting that Chatterjee (1973) and Chatterjee *et al.* (1975) observed certain relationships between histamine formation and

Table 4.2. Distribution of ascorbate in bovine eyes (mg ascorbate per kilo wet weight of tissue)

Eye tissue	Sclera	Vitreous body	Choroid and tapetum	Aqueous humour	Retina	Iris	Ciliary body	Cornea	Lens	Corneal epithelium
Ascorbate	50	150	150	190*	220	240	300	300	340	470–940†

* Heath *et al.* (1961).
† Pirie (1946).

influence and ascorbate, and that oral administration of 500 mg of vitamin C reduced the airway-constrictor effects induced by inhalation of histamine or by its release (Zuskin *et al.*, 1973). Also, Dawson and West (1965) noted that ascorbic acid has some antihistamine activity.

4.5. Eye-lens and ascorbate activity

Overall the eye contains significantly more ascorbate than plasma. However, the distribution of ascorbate varies from species to species, and particularly in the various constituent tissues of the eye and with age (e.g. Nordmann and Wien, 1934). The variation of ascorbate distribution in eye constituents can be illustrated by reference to the bovine eye; see Table 4.2.

It is characteristic of the human eye lens which has acquired cataract that the ascorbate content is very much lower than that of the normal eye. This can be appreciated from Table 4.3.

Table 4.3. Ascorbate distribution in normal and cataractous human eye lenses (mg ascorbate per kilo of wet tissue)

Eye-lens	Mean ascorbate concentration		
	Young	Adult	Mean
Normal	298*	199*	310†
Cataractous			55*
			0–5†

* Bietti (1935).
† von Euler and Malmberg (1936).

In the present state of knowledge it is difficult to specify a precise function in which the comparatively high concentrations of ascorbate in the eye-lens are involved. It is however relevant that the emergence of a cataractous state in the eye-lens is accompanied by a significant decrease in sulphydryl group concentration (e.g. Dische and Zil, 1951). It has already been pointed out that high nascent ascorbate free-radical concentrations are likely to be helpful in reduction of disulphide groups and that ascorbate opposes the oxidation of −SH groups by oxidants such as adrenochrome, and is also required for biosynthesis of −SH/−SS− containing proteins. It is therefore quite possible that the decrease in ascorbate concentration in the eye-lens (which may arise from decreased active transport, from too low an intake or from increased deactivation) is respon-sible—at any rate in part—for failing to suppress the development of cataract.

4.6. Brain tissue and ascorbate activity

The ascorbate concentrations in various parts of the brain—and by inference those in nervous tissue in general—are quite high, but they decrease with age. Thus, Schaus (1957) noted a decrease from c. 452 mg ascorbate to c. 103 mg ascorbate (per kilo of wet human cerebral tissue) from birth to over 80 years of age). Plaut and Bülow (1935) noted decreases from 650 to 75, from 370 to 90 and from 160 to 110 mg ascorbate per kilo of wet tissue over the age-span from fetuses (3–5 months) to old people (65 to 82 years old) for the cerebral cortex, cerebellar cortex and spinal cord respectively. (For additional references, see Kirk, 1962.) Melka (1936) obtained respec-tively for the cerebellum and the cerebrum averages of 260 and 160 mg per kilo wet tissue.

In order to appreciate the significance of the comparatively high ascorbate concentrations, it is helpful to consider briefly the mechan-ism of nervous transmission, and of ascorbate contribution to its efficient operation; this is presented in section 4.10.2. On that basis ascorbate is required in
  (i) the process of formation of the neurotransmitters nor-adrenaline and serotonin,
 (ii) protective association with noradrenaline, and
(iii) reduction of any noradrenochrome formed (particularly when excess leakage takes place) so that its toxic effects as well as interference with acetylcholine-esterase are inhibited.

It follows that the greater the mental stress conditions to which individuals are subjected—see section 4.10—the greater is the require-ment for ascorbate and correspondingly the greater should be the quantity of ascorbate stored.

4.7. Pancreatic tissue and ascorbate utilization

The concentration of ascorbate in the pancreas has been deter-mined by Yavorsky et al. (1934); it was found to decrease from 365, 304, 225, 152 to 95 mg (per kilo of wet tissue) for babies (1 to 30 days old), infants (1 to 12 months old), children (1 to 10 years old), adolescents/adults (11 to 45 years old), and adults/aged (47 to 77 years) respectively.

The islets of Langerhans (i.e. the β-cells) of the pancreas are responsible for the formation of pro-insulin (which subsequently matures to insulin by scission of the C-peptide) which contains a number of disulphide bonds; and on the basis of the outline given in section 4.4.2 it is to be expected that ascorbate may be utilized in this connection. However, another important function can be reasonably ascribed to the ascorbate present in this tissue, namely participation in the maintenance of physiological levels of cyclic AMP and cyclic GMP in the system. Tissues which are particularly rich in cyclic AMP can reasonably be expected to be associated with high ascorbate content (see section 4.9). The findings of Turtle and Kipnis (1968) that the islets of Langerhans of rat pancreas contain remarkably high levels of cyclic AMP are consistent with the pattern proposed here. It is worthwhile emphasizing that the ascorbate content evaluated for the pancreas as a whole may well fall short of that in the islets of Langerhans. A comparison of the values prevailing in the α-cells and β-cells is therefore desirable since this should correlate with their different functions (production of proteolytic enzymes and proinsulin).

4.8. Direct biological activities of ascorbate

It is worthwhile emphasizing that ascorbate can exert biological effects by virtue of both direct and indirect activities.

In direct activities, the result is directly connected with the presence of the ascorbate. In indirect activities the ascorbate affects the structure of, or the concentration levels of, another substance which in turn gives rise to particular physiological effects. Examples of direct activities are: the dissolution of arterial deposits, the excretion of partner-cation of the ascorbate, association of phosphodiesterase with ascorbate resulting in adverse effects on the hydrolysis of c-AMP by PDE. Examples of indirect activities are the enhancement of formation of c-AMP and corresponding physiological effects and the ascorbate-mediated catalysis of the formation of noradrenaline and adrenaline, the latter activating adenylate-cyclase to potentiate formation of c-AMP from ATP.

4.8.1. Dissolution of arterial deposits

Arterial "furry" deposits can be described as insoluble complexes of calcium/phospholipid/cholesterol. Such complexes can be dissolved by increasing concentrations of ascorbate. I have noted that aged artificial precipitates of such deposits (made by mixing individual solutions of calcium salts, phospholipids and cholesterol and allowing them to age) tend to be re-dissolved by shaking vigorously with large volumes of sodium ascorbate/physiological saline solutions which contain >20 mg ascorbate per 100 ml.

The results are in accord with the proposed suggestion (Lewin, 1974b) that higher ascorbate concentrations in the serum would tend to re-dissolve the furry arterial deposits by two complementary activities, namely:

(i) some lowering of the surface tension of the serum with consequent enhancement of the removal of the cholesterol* constituent from the arterial deposits, and

(ii) removal of the calcium from the arterial deposits, thus

$$2 \text{ Ascorbate}^- \text{ Na}^+ + \left\{ \begin{array}{c} \text{Ca}^{++}, 2 \text{ (phospholipid)} \\ \text{cholesterol} \end{array} \right\} \rightleftharpoons$$

Insoluble

$$2 \text{ Ascorbate}^-, \text{Ca}^{++} + 2 \text{ Na}^+ \text{ phospholipid}^-$$

Soluble   Soluble

4.8.2. Removal of cations

Intake of large quantities of ascorbic *acid* can be computed to enhance removal of Na^{++} via the urine, thereby reducing the level of sodium ions in the serum, as follows.

The pH value of urine in humans varies between 4.6 and 8.2 with an average cluster of values at about pH 6 (e.g. Pitts *et al.*, 1948; Smith, 1951; Schwab and Kuhns, 1959; Consolazio *et al.*, 1960). At this pH value vitamin C is almost entirely in the singly charged anionic form, accompanied by a positive counterion; and this applies to the excreted material. Most of the cations excreted in the urine are metallic, with Na^+ forming the highest concentration. It can be computed that when about 3 g of vitamin C are excreted in the urine, about 0.4 g of additional Na^+ should be co-excreted, thereby

---

* The solubility of cholesterol rises with decrease in the surface tension of the solvent medium. The surface tension of serum/air at 37°C is *c*. 47 dyn/cm (Lewin, 1972). The presence of ascorbic acid/ascorbate lowers the surface tension of water/air by over 20 dyn/cm (e.g. Künzel, 1941) and that of serum/air by several dynes.

benefiting patients in which the level of Na^+ should be lowered (e.g. patients with coronary malfunction).*

It should be noted that in addition to enhanced excretion of Na^+, enhanced excretion of K^+, NH_4^+, Ca^{++}, Mg^{++}, iron, copper and zinc is to be expected although to a much lower extent. The latter enhancement is currently being monitored in a number of volunteers. Further, the highly toxic Pb^{++}, Hg^{++}, Cd^{++} and radioactive Sr^{++} should also display enhanced excretion. Experimental evidence exists (Ruskin and Ruskin, 1952; Gontzea et al., 1963; Marchmont-Robinson, 1941) that the intake of meta quantities of vitamin C results in amelioration and increased resistance to the toxic effects following ingestion of mercury and lead; this could be due, at least in part, to increased removal as cationic partners of the ascorbate anion in the urine, and possibly also to removal by precipitation (e.g. on reduction, thus Hg^{++} (soluble) $\rightarrow Hg^+$ (insoluble)), which is thereby inhibited from interfering with biologically essential SH groups.

It has been suggested that high intake of ascorbic acid may actually enhance intestinal absorption of toxic metals such as Hg and Pb (Sahagian et al., 1967; Grimble and Hughes, 1967). However the reducing properties of high concentrations of ascorbate should, when taken orally, exert an opposing influence by tending to form the reduced—precipitable—forms of Hg^{++} and Pb^{++} within the intestines (or even in the stomach) thereby enhancing their excretion in the faeces.

4.8.3. Detoxifying activity of ascorbic acid on nitrosamines

Nitrosamines are formed by the action of nitrites on a variety of amines at the pH range of the mammalian stomach to yield toxic nitrosamines (e.g. Lijinsky and Greenblatt, 1972). This activity was found to be prevented by ascorbic acid in experiments on rats (Kamm et al., 1973). To be effective the acid must be present along with the material producing the nitrosamines at 70 mg per kilogram body weight (i.e. 5 g per 70 g body weight) and above to prevent liberation of the nitrosamine into the serum. For discussion of possible mechanisms see Walters (1974).

---

* Increased uptake of ascorbic *acid* results in decreased pH values of the urine (pH < 6). Hence, considerable increase in the amount of the acid consumed does not result in corresponding increase in excretion of Na^+ (see also McDonald and Murphy, 1959).

4.8.4. Biosynthetic activities

Ascorbate is implicated—probably via its free radical—in various enzymatically controlled activities which range widely from the formation of γ-globulins to general hydroxylation activities such as those participating in the formation of collagen (hydroxyproline and hydroxylysine), noradrenaline and tryptophan-5-hydroxylase.

γ-Globulins. Biosynthesis of γ-globulins—as in leucocytes—has already been considered in section 4.4.2. The principles outlined there are applicable to the formation of other proteins with disulphide bridges.

Formation of noradrenaline and adrenaline. Outlines of the formation of noradrenaline and of adrenaline have been presented in section 4.3.1, while complementary H... bonding and molecular model construction considerations in favour of formation of noradrenaline-ascorbate and adrenaline-ascorbate (useful for protective purposes) have been considered in section 1.2.8.3. It is relevant that an AFR signal has been observed in a complete incubation medium in which dopamine β-hydroxylose catalyses the conversion of dopamine to noradrenaline (Blumberg *et al.*, 1965).

Formation of collagen. Considerable evidence is available that ascorbate is essential for the hydroxylation of the proline and lysine required in the formation of collagen; for a comprehensive review see Barnes and Kodicek (1972). Active hydroxyl radicals may well arise from the intervention of the ascorbic free radical. Evidence has been obtained (Gould, 1970) in favour of folate-ascorbate interactions in collagen formation.

4.9. Indirect biological influence of ascorbate on cyclic nucleotide-mediated hormonal activities

Many physiological activities are potentiated by hormonal actions which utilize cyclic AMP and cyclic GMP as "Second Messengers" or mediators. The activities of the cyclic nucleotides extend to many physiological fields; and the extent of their activities depends on their respective concentration levels. It follows that if ascorbate enhances higher concentration levels of these nucleotides, it can be considered to have an effect—albeit indirectly—on the particular physiological activity. In this connection I shall develop a pattern which traces the activity of ascorbate in maintaining the necessary concentration levels of both cyclic AMP and cyclic GMP.*

However, before proceeding with this, it is useful to outline very briefly the physiological potential of c-AMP and c-GMP.

4.9.1. Maintenance of physiological actions by c-AMP and c-GMP

The concept that c-AMP acts as a mediator or "Second Messenger" in respect of hormonal activities was proposed and established by Sutherland and his co-workers (for references see Robison, Butcher and Sutherland, 1971; Major and Kilpatrick, 1972). The following table which gives several—but by no means all—physiological activities in which c—AMP has been shown to participate should enable appreciation of the wide extent of its involvement.

Table 4.4. Hormonal activities in which c-AMP is involved

Hormone	c-AMP involvement in
Adrenaline	Glycolysis; heart contraction; stimulation of enzyme secretions; lipolysis of fat cells; β-insulin secretion; β-melanophore stimulation
ACTH	Phosphorylase activation; protein kinase activation; steroid synthesis; lipolysis of fat cells
LH	Glucose uptake; glycolysis; steroid synthesis
TSH	Thyroid growth and cell division; release of thyroid hormones; phosphorylase activity; glucose uptake
Vasopressin	Transport of H_2O, Na^+ and urea
Oxytocin	Enzyme secretion
Glucagon	Glycolysis; heart contraction; transport of K^+ and urea

It is difficult to see how the wide extent of c-AMP influence can achieve specificity of action. Indeed, the type of action which it exercises is determined by the enzymatic profile of the cell in which the action takes place. It is not apposite to consider at this stage various activities of c-AMP in detail; but, as an example of its activity

---

* The proposal (Lewin, 1973, 1974) that ascorbate contributes to the maintenance of physiological c-AMP levels via adrenaline formation (and subsequent activation of adenylcyclase) and via the inhibition of PDE has been experimentally substantiated by Van Wyk and Kotzé (1975) who found that the administration of ascorbate to baboons resulted in 30 to 40% rise in c-AMP and c-GMP content of the blood, and by Tisdale (1975) who reported that ascorbate inhibits PDE activity.

on different tissues we can draw attention to the effect on cholesterol. C-AMP inhibits the conversion of acetate to cholesterol in liver (Berthet, 1960). Also, in the adrenal cortex, the corpus leuteum, the ovary and testis increased levels of c-AMP stimulate the conversion of cholesterol to progenenolone. Thus increased levels of c-AMP should favour lower cholesterol levels. Indeed, some investigators have observed reduced cholesterol levels subsequent to mega intake of vitamin C; see Table 7.2.

4.9.2. The link between ascorbate and c-AMP and c-GMP

4.9.2.1. *Outline of the concept*

First, a number of experimental/clinical data will be given showing a parallelism between ascorbate and c-AMP activities and of coincident involvement of c-GMP; also experimental evidence will be presented showing that ascorbate affects adversely the hydrolytical breakdown of c-AMP by phosphodiesterase (PDE) and thereby enhances higher concentration levels of c-AMP.

Second, a scheme will be presented showing how ascorbate is responsible for processes which contribute not only to formation of c-AMP but also to inhibition of processes which reduce the concentration levels of c-AMP and c-GMP by hydrolysing them to 5'AMP and 5'GMP respectively.

Third, a number of physiological activities which are mediated by the two cyclic nucleotides (to which higher concentrations of vitamin C are likely to contribute) will be traced, although the experimental link may not as yet have been reported.

4.9.2.2. *Co-presence and coincident activities of ascorbate and of c-AMP and c-GMP*

(i) *Cancer*. Ascorbate was found to be highly toxic to Erhlich ascites-carcinoma cells (Benade *et al.*, 1969). Ascorbate concentrations are depleted in malignant activity (see, for example, Waldo and Zipf, 1955); diminished adenyl cyclase activity has been noted in polyoma-virus-transformed cells (Bürk, 1968). Tumour growth was inhibited by c-AMP (Gericke and Chandra, 1969). Cell growth *in vitro* can be inhibited by c-AMP (Ryan and Heidrick, 1968); thymic lymphocytes are inhibited by high concentrations of c-AMP, $>10^{-4}$ M (MacManus and Whitfield, 1969).

(ii) *ACTH*. In general, cortex c-AMP has been shown to mimic the effects of ACTH on ascorbate depletion (Earp *et al.*, 1969, 1970).

(iii) *Pancreas*. High concentrations of ascorbate have been found in the pancreas (Yavorsky *et al.*, 1934; see also Table 4.1). High concentrations of c-AMP have been found in the islets of Langerhan (Turtle and Kipnis, 1967).

(iv) *Antiviral activity*. Viral infection may be counteracted by interferon. The presence of 1 mM c-AMP results in significant antiviral activity in chicken fibroblasts by virtue of interferon formation; this contrasts with the absence of antiviral activity by c-AMP alone, and with the inability of 5'AMP to potentiate interferon activity (Friedman and Pastan, 1969). Symptoms of Herpes (cold-sore) virus are suppressed by mega intake of ascorbic acid (see section 7.7.3).

(v) *c-AMP and c-GMP involvement with insulin and ascorbate in respect of hypoglycemia*.

(a) *Insulin and ascorbate*. High intake of vitamin C parallels insulin activity in tending to result in lower blood sugar levels. Several workers have shown that intravenous intake of the vitamin (in the region of 0.3 to 1.2 gm) results in significant lowering of the blood sugar curves in normal and in diabetic patients (e.g. Secher, 1942; Sylvest, 1942). Pfleger and Scholl (1937) and Bartelheimer (1939) noted that high intake of ascorbic acid resulted in a decrease of the required insulin dose in several diabetic patients; and Dice and Daniel (1973) concluded that in one diabetic patient each gram of the vitamin C taken resulted in a decrease of the insulin dose required by 2 I.U.

(b) *C-AMP and c-GMP and insulin*. c-AMP is known to enhance insulin release from the pancreatic islets (Sussman and Vaughan, 1967; Malaisse *et al.*, 1967). Insulin adversely affects c-AMP concentrations (Senft *et al.*, 1968). Very high c-AMP concentrations are found in the pancreatic islets of rats (Turtle and Kipnis, 1967). Insulin potentiates c-GMP in adipose and in liver cells (Illiano *et al.*, 1973). c-AMP and c-GMP are mutually antagonistic (Goldberg *et al.*, 1973).

4.9.2.3. *Ascorbate and cyclic AMP* *

Adrenaline synthesis and subsequent formation of cyclic AMP. Ascorbate assists the production of adrenaline from dopamine. This

---

* A preliminary communication concerning *part* of the scheme was given at the 545th Meeting of the Biochemical Society 18–19 December, 1973 (Lewin, 1974c).

activity can be represented schematically as in Fig. 4.1. The subsequent stages concerned with formation of cyclic AMP are depicted in Fig. 4.3.

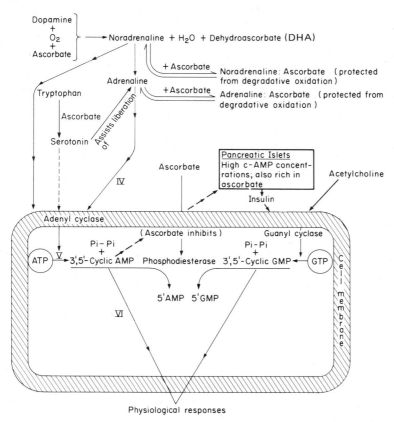

Fig. 4.3. Schematic representation of the ascorbate-enhanced formations and increased activities of c-AMP and c-GMP and associated physiological effects.

Stage I. Ascorbate or catechol is required as a co-factor by dopamine β-hydroxylase in the formation of noradrenaline from dopamine (Levin and Kaufman, 1961).

Stage II. Adrenaline is formed from noradrenaline by methylation. A limited concentration of noradrenaline-methyl-transferase could restrict synthesis of adrenaline, but ascorbate may also be utilized in this stage since Kirshner and Goodall (1957) utilized reduced gluthathione in their preparations; and reducing thiol activity can be replaced by ascorbate (see Price, 1966).

Stage III. Protection of adrenaline in the reduced 3'-4'-dihydroxy state. Under physiological conditions adrenaline can be oxidized rapidly to adrenochrome which is highly toxic. However, ascorbate rapidly reduces the oxidized compound to the reduced state. Earlier (Figs 1.7a and 1.7b), the association of ascorbate with adrenaline— via the 3'-4'-hydroxy groups—was considered to be stereochemically and energetically feasible; such association should protect adrenaline from oxidation. Indeed, experimental evidence indicates that adrenaline-ascorbate solutions are less prone to oxidative attack (Beauvillain and Sarradin, 1948).

Adrenaline potentiates the adenyl cyclase in the membrane (Stage IV shown in Fig. 4.3) which in turn activates the formation of cyclic AMP from ATP (Stage V is shown in Fig. 4.3).

The *last two stages* have been considered in the literature; for extensive reference and tabulation see Robison *et al.* (1971). It is proposed here that the adrenaline-ascorbate complex activates adenylcyclase on release of the adrenaline or possibly even directly. In the latter case the 3'- and 4'-hydroxy groups of the adrenaline would be masked.

Inhibition of the hydrolytic activity of PDE on cyclic AMP. PDE hydrolyses cyclic AMP (Stage VII shown in Fig. 4.3). It is indicative that cyclic AMP and ascorbate each possesses a ring-structure with a negatively charged oxygen. This parallelism and the production of an acid group, when each ring is hydrolysed, suggest the possibility that ascorbate would compete with cyclic AMP for the enzyme's active sites when the two are present in a total quantity sufficient to saturate the PDE, thereby causing decreased hydrolysis of cyclic AMP. Indeed, Moffat *et al.* (1972) have shown that L-ascorbate is effective in concentrations as low as 10^{-4} M in inhibiting the breakdown of c-AMP. I have confirmed these observations at 0.8×10^{-4} M ascorbate and also the conclusion that L-ascorbate completes with c-AMP for PDE, using the pH statting method. I have also followed the hydrolysis of ascorbate by PDE using pH statting (see section 3.3.2).

Activity of c-AMP in relation to PDE and ascorbate. Cyclic AMP potentiates hormonal actions, synthesis of a number of enzymes and of several physiological activities in proportion to its concentration. For original references see Table 5.1 in Robison *et al.*, 1971.

As can be appreciated from Fig. 4.3, the concentration level of c-AMP depends on its formation and destruction, in

    (i) activation of formation from ATP following adenylcyclase activity which in turn is potentiated by adrenaline, and

(ii) reduction of the activity of PDE which catalyses hydrolysis to 5'AMP (see above section).

Cellular concentrations of cyclic AMP can vary from $c.$ 10^{-6} to 10^{-4} M. If the cellular ascorbate ion concentration can reach these or higher levels, it is likely to compete effectively with and displace cyclic AMP from the active sites in PDE, thus tending to inhibit hydrolysis of cyclic AMP and preventing reduction in its concentration. Now, intake of mega quantities of vitamin C has been shown by several workers to raise the levels of ascorbate concentration in the blood from $c.$ 0.8 mg to $c.$ 2.4 mg per 100 ml of blood.* An average value of 2 mg of ascorbate per 100 ml of serum would be equivalent to over 10^{-4} M ascorbate. However, the concentration of ascorbate in the serum is representative only of the *lowest* values, because ascorbate transfer mechanisms exist in various tissues resulting in corresponding increases in ascorbate concentration. It has been established by numerous investigators that many tissues have much higher ascorbate levels. For several references see Tables 4.1, 4.2 and 4.3. It is therefore reasonable to postulate that the higher concentrations of ascorbate will result in increased interaction with PDE thereby reducing the latter's association with cyclic AMP and consequent rescue from being hydrolysed to 5'AMP, thus allowing cyclic AMP concentrations to rise, on being formed from ATP. The following experimental findings are in accord with this proposed pattern.

Higher cellular concentrations of cyclic AMP are reflected in increased concentrations in the urine. Thus, Broadus *et al.* (1970) found that infusion of adrenaline raises the cyclic AMP levels in both plasma and urine; and Owen and Moffat (personal communication) noted over 30% increase in the level of cyclic AMP excreted in the urine following several days of daily intake of 2 g of ascorbic acid. See also footnote relating to section 4.9.

Cyclic GMP: Formation of cyclic GMP, its competitive association with PDE and resultant hydrolysis to 5'GMP. When guanyl cyclase is activated by certain hormones (which do not include adrenaline) GTP is potentiated to form cyclic GMP and pyrophosphate. Ascorbate does not appear to assist hormones which potentiate guanyl cyclase directly or indirectly—via surface receptors—as is the case with

---

* Different workers give different values: e.g. Masek and Hruba (1964), Kübler and Gehler (1970), Spero (1973), and Coulehan (1974); but in general there is agreement that increase in vitamin C intake results in higher *blood* content of ascorbate which tails off due to renal threshold. As will be outlined in Chapter 6, increase in absorption of ascorbate by the tissues continues in spite of the steady state of concentration attained by the blood.

insulin. However, the anionic cyclic GMP, being identical with that in cyclic AMP, is also similar to the anionic section in ascorbate.

Now, it has been established that cyclic GMP and cyclic AMP can be hydrolysed by a single phosphodiesterase (Beavo *et al.*, 1970); also that cyclic GMP can be a competitive inhibitor of cyclic AMP (Goren *et al.*, 1970). In normal physiological conditions cyclic GMP need not compete with cyclic AMP (for association with PDE) and thereby save it from hydrolysis, and vice versa, because the respective concentrations (allowing for their respective association constant values with PDE) are insufficient to saturate PDE. However, as the ascorbate concentration in the tissues is raised on increased absorption, following intake of mega quantities of the vitamin, increased association with the active sites in PDE should take place, thereby leaving correspondingly smaller numbers of sites for association with cyclic AMP and cyclic GMP. It is now that the competition between the two cyclonucleotides—for the few remaining active sites in PDE—should become prominent, thereby favouring their physiological "mutual antagonism" recently propounded in the literature (Goldberg *et al.*, 1973). Perhaps the major significance of this aspect lies in the indications that particular balanced concentration ratios of {[cyclic AMP]/[cyclic GMP]} may control some types of malignant tissue development more effectively than cyclic AMP alone (Ryan and Heidrick, 1968) without adversely affecting physiologically essential activities.

In this connection it is relevant that the two cyclic nucleotides can compete for one particular binding protein. Indeed, Crozier *et al.* (1974) have concluded, using cyclic AMP binding proteins from bovine adrenal glands, that c-GMP can displace c-AMP from its association with the binding proteins. It is reasonable to expect that ascorbate will exert some displacing action to displace both cyclic nucleotides from their association with these binding proteins.

4.10. Ascorbate and control of physiological activities

4.10.1. Ascorbate influence on formation of hormones

We have seen that the formation of the hormones noradrenaline, adrenaline and serotonin (see section 2.3.2.5) are influenced by ascorbate, and that c-AMP and c-GMP concentration levels are also affected by ascorbate. It is worthwhile stressing that c-AMP acts not only as a second messenger mediating hormonal actions, but also exerts influence on the formation of hormones, as can be appreciated from Table 4.4. Because ascorbate is able to increase the levels of c-AMP and c-GMP, it should be able to influence—although indirectly—the formation of several other hormones besides nor-adrenaline, adrenaline and serotonin. However, this effect may be missed unless note is taken of the various infeeds and feedbacks in which the cyclic nucleotides are involved.

From what has been said in Chapters 1 and 2, it should be clear that ascorbate is capable of influencing several other participating activities. To cover all these influences in detail would require a tome; obviously this cannot be carried out in the space available here.

4.10.2. Ascorbate influence on neuro-transmission

In this section we shall consider the effect ascorbate can be expected to have on activities of nervous transmission. It is generally accepted that the nervous system uses, for mediation of the nervous impulse, primarily the two neuro-transmitters noradrenaline and acetylcholine, and that serotonin is most likely a neuro-humoral transmitter in the "tryptaminergic" nerves in mammals (Brodie and Costa, 1962). Nervous transmission involves the release of the neurotransmitter at the synapse, that is at the junction of the two nerves along which the neural message travels, or where it is to be delivered. Deactivation of the neuro-transmitters follows: nor-adrenaline is degraded, while acetylcholine is hydrolysed by the enzyme acetylcholine-esterase, and—where effective—serotonin is deactivated by oxidative deamination. Deactivation is essential so that the nervous impulse is conveyed only when it is impelled, and is terminated once the source which triggers the message is no longer active; were it not so, the liberated neuro-transmitter would persist in its activity long after cessation of the induction of the original message. The neuro-transmitters are impelled when the nervous impulse is operative, and of necessity they must be synthesized/ stored for use as required. It follows that malfunctions of nervous operations can arise if the mechanism of deactivation is faulty, or if the toxic noradrenochrome and adrenochrome are not rapidly neutralized.

The pattern which I have developed at the molecular level, of the various clinical physiological observations encompassing mega-intake of vitamin C with enhancement of formation of the neuro-trans-mitters, lessening of noradrenochrome formation, and raising of both cyclic AMP and cyclic GMP levels collates various relevant experimental findings, thus:

Collation of low vitamin C levels, low cyclic AMP levels, and depressed mental levels. Individuals with depressed mental states have lower serum vitamin C levels (e.g. Milner, 1963; Punekar, 1961) as well as low cyclic AMP levels (e.g. Paul *et al.*, 1970, 1971; Abdulla and Hamadah, 1970; Ramsden, 1970).

Collation of raised vitamin C levels and raised cyclic nucleotide levels with mental therapy. Therapeutic effect is experienced by individuals in mentally depressed states; including schizophrenia— when they follow a regime of mega-intake of ascorbic acid (e.g. Vander Kamp, 1966). High intake of vitamin C results in higher tissue absorption, despite the steady state levels attained by serum (e.g. Kubler and Gehler, 1970).

High tissue ascorbate levels enhance higher levels of availability of

(i) *noradrenaline*, by direct production and indirectly by protection from early degradation while being formed (Fig. 4.1), and

(ii) *Cyclic AMP*: noradrenaline (or adrenaline) activate adenylcyclase which in turn potentiates formation of cyclic AMP (Lewin, 1973) as well as inactivation of phosphodiesterase (Moffat *et al.*, 1972), the enzyme which is responsible for hydrolytic breakdown of cyclic purine nucleotides. This is borne out by the finding that intake of daily multigrams of vitamin C results in increased cyclic AMP levels in serum, evidenced in turn by greater daily urinary excretion of cyclic AMP (Owen and Moffat, 1974, personal communication; see also footnote to section 4.9). Inhibition of the enzyme also results in raised levels of cyclic *GMP* (e.g. Beavo *et al.*, 1970; Goren *et al.*, 1970).

The overall scheme is represented in Fig. 4.3.

Evidence exists of an inter-relationship between acetylcholine and cyclic nucleotide levels. Acetylcholine is responsible for an increase in cyclic GMP levels and a decrease in cyclic AMP levels (for several references and useful discussion see Robison *et al.*, 1971). Abnormal acetylcholine activity could therefore result in lowering of cyclic AMP levels to an undesirable extent; this would be compensated for by the presence of high ascorbate levels tending to raise the cyclic AMP levels.

This scheme incorporates a safety aspect in respect of formation of higher than normal cyclic AMP levels. High levels of ascorbate result in higher levels of *both* cyclic AMP and cyclic GMP. The two nucleotides are mutually antagonistic (Goldberg *et al.*, 1973) thereby affording protection from too high cyclic AMP levels which on their own could enhance manic states.

4.11. Indirect detoxifying activity of ascorbate on nerve depressants (such as barbitals) and carcinogenic substances (such as chloretone)

Animals capable of synthesizing their own vitamin C requirements have been shown, when exposed to intake of nerve depressants (such as barbitals) and carcinogenic agents (such as chloretone) to increase their vitamin C biosynthesis multifold (e.g. Longenecker *et al.*, 1939, 1940; Evans *et al.*, 1960). High intake of ascorbate was also shown to exert a protective influence against normally lethal doses (Einhauser, 1939).

The respective mechanisms of carcinogenic compounds are not known with certainty. However, the enhancing effect of barbital on the formation of intermediate steps in ascorbate biosynthesis has been elucidated (see section 5.3.2). It is quite probable that nerve depressants act partly by depressing c-AMP levels, and that the protective influence of ascorbate against lethal doses of barbital is due to the tendency to counteract this depression. This possibility is supported by my findings (carried out on eight individuals) that intake of 1 g ascorbic acid with sodium amytal (60 grains to 160 grains) at night reduces the sedative tendency as compared to the times when sodium amytal alone was taken.

4.12. *Modus operandi* of DHA

4.12.1. Overview of direct activities

DHA possesses five biologically significant abilities (see also sections 1.3.6.1 and 1.3.6.2):
(a) Penetration of cellular membranes (walls);
(b) reduction to ascorbate;
(c) oxidation to 2:3-diketogluconate;
(d) combination with amino/imino groups or sulphydryl groups; and
(e) opening of its γ-lactone structure by hydrolysis (Kagawa and Takiguchi, 1961; Kawada *et al.*, 1962).

The first characteristic is useful in transporting the ascorbic system into cells (since ascorbate has only slight membrane-penetrating power) provided DHA can be rapidly reduced within the cell to ascorbate.

These characteristics are competitive. Thus, so far as the −SH groups are concerned.

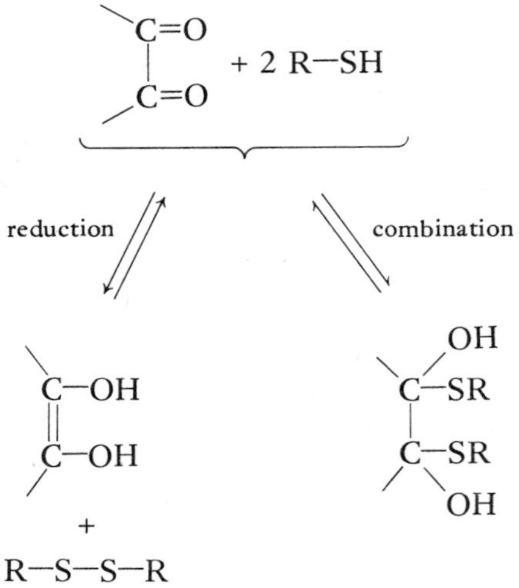

$$
\begin{array}{c}
\backslash C=O \\
| \\
{}_{\diagup} C=O
\end{array}
\quad + 2\ R{-}SH
$$

reduction   combination

$$
\begin{array}{c}
\backslash C{-}OH \\
\| \\
{}_{\diagup} C{-}OH
\end{array}
\qquad
\begin{array}{c}
OH \\
\backslash \diagup \\
C{-}SR \\
| \\
C{-}SR \\
\diagup \backslash \\
OH
\end{array}
$$

+

R−S−S−R

The ability to be reduced to ascorbate is part of the biological redox activities of the ascorbic system which are physiologically essential. However, the ability to combine reversibly with −SH groups to form the corresponding OH derivative results in unavailability of the DHA for the usual redox activities. Also, excessive removal of −SH groups from the biological medium enhances deactivation of numerous enzymes which depend on the −SH group for their activities. Hence, high DHA concentrations can be expected to be deleterious to a number of biological activities. It is therefore not surprising to find special enzymes which are engaged in catalysing the reduction of DHA to AA by the use of free (unattached) glutathione (e.g. Christine et al., 1956) thus sparing −SH groups of enzymes. It is also known experimentally that DHA can adversely affect health. Thus, Patterson (1950) found that DHA is diabetogenic. The hydrolysis of the γ-lactone ring could be considered physiologically disadvantageous, since the resulting products can no longer be reversibly reformed into DHA, and sooner or later can end up in oxalic acid (a physiologically deleterious compound) or in L-lyxonic acid and L-xylose (see Fig. 1.4).

4.12.2. Possible participation of AA/DHA in mitotic control

It was observed by Stern and Timonen (1954) that nuclei of calf-thymus and liver contain not only high concentrations of reduced glutathione but also comparatively high concentrations of ascorbate (the latter being equivalent to $c.$ 1.62 and 1.41 g AA per kilo of the respective tissues); and further, that in lily anthers the concentration of AA rises to a maximum value during mitosis $c.$ 2.2 g per kilo) but is much lowered when mitosis is over. These observations and those of Price (1966) that ascorbate addition enhances RNA synthesis in wheat nuclei support the notion that ascorbate participates in the activity of the nucleus in respect of both mitotic activity and RNA transcription.

Szent Györgyi (1968) advocated that cell division could be controlled by the mutual antagonism of two substances namely a promoter ("promine") and an inhibitor ("retine"). He further suggested that the glyoxalase enzyme system could act as a promoter, while the inhibitor may be an electron acceptor possessing a glyoxal group. Edgar (1969) argued that DHA could act as an inhibitor representing retine, and that a possible role for ascorbic acid would be to maintain the level of DHA in the tumour-inhibiting effect.

However, in view of the pattern developed here earlier on and later on, of the various direct and indirect activities of the ascorbic system including AFR, cyclic nucleotides and other factors, it is rather difficult to escape the conclusion that Szent-Györgyi's (1968) suggestion is an over-simplification of the potential of the interplay of mitotic and RNA translational activities of the chromatin; and further that Edgar's suggestion (1969) may well be an approach in which cause and effect are confused in that AA and AFR could be more appropriately described as the driving and energy-transporting entities, while DHA is a product which can cause more adverse as well as beneficial activities, and that DHA's main biological uses are the ability to cross wall-membranes and thereafter be transformed into ascorbate.

Chapter 5

Biosynthesis and metabolism

5.1. Biosynthetic ability and siting

Understanding of the inability of humans and of other animals to meet, by biosynthesis, their own needs of ascorbic acid, and of the effect thereon of possible genetic variations under "normal" conditions and under biochemical stress, requires an outline of the biosynthetic paths and metabolic activity of the vitamin.

The results of numerous published investigations* on the biosynthesis of ascorbic acid may be conveniently summarized as follows:

Ascorbic acid participates in the metabolism of living organisms, whether biosynthesized by the organism or obtained exogenously from the diet. All chlorophyl-containing plants appear capable of biosynthesizing ascorbic acid. Not all members of the animal kingdom appear capable of expressing the *entire* sequence of operational steps required in the biosynthesis. Further, the site of biosynthesis of ascorbic acid while located mainly† in the microsomal fractions, has been shown to be restricted to the *liver and/or the kidney* in the respective animals. In general, invertebrates, insects and fishes, flying mammals (e.g. *Pteropus medius* and *Vasperugo abramus*), many primates, the guinea pig, and birds of higher orders (the Passeres) appear unable to biosynthesize the vitamin; whereas amphibians, reptiles and lower order birds have been found to biosynthesize the vitamin in the kidney. Also, the more evolved birds (Passeriformas)

---

* E.g. Burns and Evans, 1956; Hassan and Lehninger, 1956; Chatterjee *et al.*, 1957; Burns, 1957; Roy and Guha, 1958; Chatterjee *et al.*, 1960; Chatterjee *et al.*, 1961; Chauduri and Chatterjee, 1969; Gupta *et al.*, 1972; Chatterjee, 1973a, b.

† There exists some evidence that not only the mitochondria of plants but also those of certain animals can participate in, and contribute to biosynthesis of ascorbate (see section 5.4).

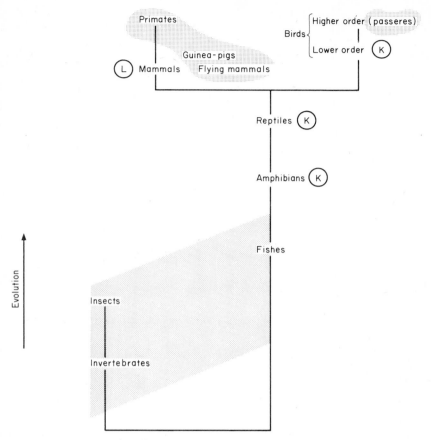

Fig. 5.1. Ability of different species of animals to biosynthesize ascorbate. Shaded areas represent defective biosynthesis. Ⓚ and Ⓛ represent respectively microsomal kidney and microsomal biosynthesis of ascorbate. (Based on Chatterjee, 1973.)

and most mammals biosynthesize ascorbic acid in the liver. The ability and siting of biosynthesis of ascorbic acid can be related to evolution schematically as is illustrated in Fig. 5.1.

5.2. Biosynthetic paths in plants

Utilizing radioactive tracer techniques, three major paths have been proposed for the biosynthesis of ascorbic acid in plants. Of these, two have been proposed by Isherwood and his co-workers while the third has been proposed by Loewus and his co-workers.

The two major biosynthetic paths proposed by Isherwood, Chen and Mapson (1954) on the basis of their work on cress seedlings will, for the sake of convenience, be termed the glucose–glucuronic-gulonic path and the galactose–galacturonate–galactonolactone path respectively. These paths involve respective inversions of C-1 of glucose and of C-1 galactose to C-6 of L-ascorbic acid, as is shown by the asterisks.

(i) *The glucose-glucuronic-gulonic path.*

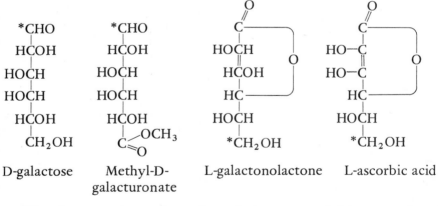

D-glucose   D-glucuronic acid   L-gulonic acid   L-ascorbic acid

(ii) *The galactose-galacturonate-galactonolactone path.*

D-galactose   Methyl-D-   L-galactonolactone   L-ascorbic acid
                   galacturonate

(iii) The experimental results of Loewus and his co-workers (Loewus *et al.*, 1956; 1957; Loewus, 1961)—using ripening strawberries and also germinating cress seedlings—do not unequivocally support the above mechanisms proposed by Isherwood and co-workers as major pathways, as comparatively little evidence for inversion between D-glucose and L-ascorbic acid was found. For example, they found that D-glucose-1-^{14}C gave ascorbic acid with

65–70% of its activity in C-1 and 14–19% in C-6; whereas using D-glucose-6-^{14}C, 73% of the total activity in the resulting ascorbic acid was found in C-6 and 24% in C-1. Using D-galactose-1-^{14}C the resulting activity in the ascorbic acid was about equally distributed between C-1 and C-6. The marked distinction between these results and those obtained in rats (where inversion of C-1 glucose and of C-1 galactose to C-6 of ascorbic acid was obtained by various workers (Jackel et al., 1950; Burns and Evans, 1956) shows that ascorbic acid biosynthetic paths in plants and animals are different.

5.3. Biosynthesis in animals

5.3.1. Outline of the biosynthetic paths

The biosynthesis of ascorbic acid in the rat has been followed by several investigators—by examining the urinary excretion of the vitamin—employing radioactive tracer techniques involving ^{14}C (Jackel et al., 1950; Horowitz et al., 1952; Horowitz and King, 1953; Isherwood et al., 1954; Burns et al., 1956; Hassan and Lehninger, 1956; Burns, 1957; Burns and Evans, 1956; Burns and Mosbach, 1956; Dayton et al., 1959; Chatterjee et al., 1958; Evans et al., 1960) D-glucose was used as the starting point, and it was established that its carbon chain is converted intact while *undergoing inversion of configuration* into L-ascorbic acid as is represented by the asterisks. The initially accepted path is given below*

| D-glucose | D-glucuronic acid | L-gulonolactone | L-ascorbic acid |

---

* In conformity with the convention in the literature, the acid forms are shown as part of the biosynthetic path. In practice the anionic forms are involved because of the neutral physiological pH range.

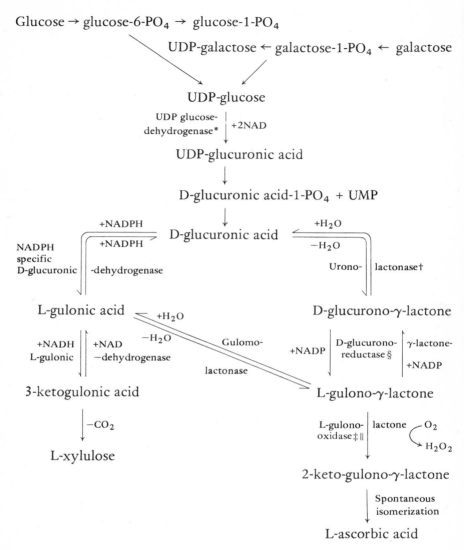

Glucose → glucose-6-PO_4 → glucose-1-PO_4

UDP-galactose ← galactose-1-PO_4 ← galactose

UDP-glucose

UDP glucose-dehydrogenase* | +2NAD

UDP-glucuronic acid

D-glucuronic acid-1-PO_4 + UMP

+NADPH   D-glucuronic acid   +H_2O

NADPH specific D-glucuronic | +NADPH -dehydrogenase   −H_2O Urono- | lactonase†

L-gulonic acid ← +H_2O D-glucurono-γ-lactone

+NADH L-gulonic | +NAD −dehydrogenase   −H_2O Gulomo-   +NADP   D-glucurono-reductase § | γ-lactone- +NADP

                                         lactonase

3-ketogulonic acid   L-gulono-γ-lactone

| −CO_2 L-gulono-oxidase‡‖ | lactone ⌒ O_2 → H_2O_2

L-xylulose

                                         2-keto-gulono-γ-lactone

                                         | Spontaneous isomerization

                                         L-ascorbic acid

* The activity of this enzyme is enhanced by chloroetone and barbitone (Touster and Holman, 1961; Conney *et al.*, 1961; Conney and Burns, 1961). See also Gupta *et al.* (1970).
† Winkelman and Lehninger (1958).
‡ Flavoprotein containing −SH groups.
§ Contains −SH groups (Chatterjee *et al.*, 1958). Cobalt acts as activator (Sasmal *et al.*, 1968).
‖ Manganese and cobalt stimulate the synthesis of L-ascorbic acid from L-gulonolactone (Sasmal *et al.*, 1968).

Fig. 5.2. The biosynthetic fork of L-ascorbic acid and L-xylulose.

Further investigations identified the intermediate steps in greater detail (e.g. Strominger *et al.*, 1954; Storey and Dutton, 1955; Evans *et al.*, 1960). Galactose was found a more effective precursor of L-ascorbic acid than D-glucose (Evans *et al.*, 1960). Further, it was shown that D-glucose is converted to D-glucuronic acid via the oxidation of uridine diphosphate-glucose to uridine-diphospho-glucuronic acid, the reaction being catalysed by an NAD-linked enzyme in the soluble fractions of the liver (Strominger *et al.*, 1954; Storey and Dutton, 1955). The results of the various investigations have led to the adoption of the following overall scheme as being the most likely (for relevant reviews see also Degkwitz *et al.*, 1964; Burns, 1967); see Fig. 5.2, where the relation of the L-xylulose biosynthetic fork is also shown.

It is apposite to consider in somewhat greater detail the later stages of Fig. 5.2, as they are likely to comprise—as will be appreciated later—the steps that are deficient in those species which are apparently unable to biosynthesize ascorbic acid.

Evidence has been gathered in favour of the pathway in which enzymes in the microsomal fractions are able to use *D-glucurono-lactone* as the substrate to L-ascorbic acid, whereas the use of *D-glucuronic acid* as a substrate requires the addition of the soluble supernatant fraction containing the enzymes necessary to convert D-glucuronic acid into L-gulonolactone, thereby allowing the micro-somes to enforce conversion into ascorbic acid (e.g. Chatterjee *et al.*, 1961; Chatterjee, 1970; Gupta *et al.*, 1970). These pathways can be schematically represented as in Fig. 5.3.

5.3.2. Effect of drugs on the biosynthesis of ascorbate

It has been established that a number of structurally different substances, such as barbiturates and halogenated aliphatic com-pounds, accelerate multifold the excretion of ascorbate in rats (e.g. Musulin *et al.*, 1938; Longenecker *et al.*, 1939; Smythe and King, 1942). The most active compounds caused the rats to excrete as much as several hundred times more vitamin C than that associated with normal diets. As the quantities excreted each day were far in excess of the total body stores—and allowing for the half life of ascorbate in the animal—the reasonable conclusion was reached that these drugs accelerate the synthesis of ascorbate and/or interfere with the metabolic paths in which it is irreversibly broken down, thereby raising the concentration level of the ascorbate, and hence its excretion. Two groups of drugs can be distinguished, namely the

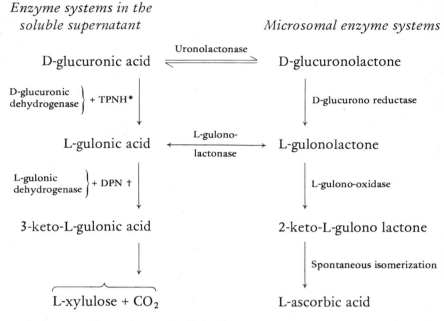

Enzyme systems in the
soluble supernatant   *Microsomal enzyme systems*

* The enzymatic reaction specifically involves TPN, thus (Bublitz *et al.*, 1958).

TPNH + D-glucuronate + H$^+$ ⇌ TPN$^+$ + L-gulonate

† This enzymatic conversion appears to require DPN, thus (Bublitz *et al.*, 1958).

L-gulonate + DPN$^+$ ⇌ 3-keto-L-gulonate + DPNH + H$^+$

Fig. 5.3. Enzyme systems in the soluble supernatant, and microsomal enzymes.

barbiturates and the halogenated hydrocarbons, and the carcinogenic hydrocarbon group (e.g. methylcholanthrene and 3,4-benzpyrene). The first group, as was pointed out by Musulin *et al.* (1938), was composed of nerve depressants.

A distinction can be drawn between the two groups in that the first group enhances the formation of UDP-glucose dehydrogenase while the second group does not appear to do so (Touster and Hollman, 1961; Conney *et al.*, 1961). An additional effect was noted by Mano *et al.* (1961) who showed that the enzyme which catalyses the conversion of D-glucuronate to L-gulonate to TPNH was inhibited specifically by barbital. From this inhibition we can infer that the increased presence of ascorbate following barbiturate intake is in part due to blocking off the L-xylulose pathway shown in Fig. 5.2, and consequent diversion of the D-glucuronic acid transformation to the ascorbic acid biosynthesis pathway. It is relevant that Gupta *et al.* (1970) have concluded that a conjugate of D-glucurono-1,4-lactone and imidazole, which is a substrate for the microsomal enzyme leading to synthesis of L-ascorbic acid, has been identified in the urine of rats treated with chloretone, barbital and 1,2-benzanthracene. Their results indicate that enhanced synthesis of L-ascorbic acid after administration of various drugs and toxic chemical compounds is due to induced formation of this endogenous substrate. While there is as yet insufficient evidence to conclude with certainty which mechanism is involved in the second group, it is apposite to note certain points in connection with the first group. Depressed mental states are known to be associated with low cyclic AMP levels (Paul *et al.*, 1970, 1971; Abdulla and Hanadah, 1970; Ramsden, 1970); hence a connection with cyclic AMP levels is indicated.

Also, since noradrenaline activity is more than likely to be lowered in depressed mental states, and since ascorbate is utilized in the formation of noradrenaline (see section 4.3), an interference with ascorbate utilization could well increase ascorbate levels. Hence part of the increased ascorbate excretion could be due to its decreased metabolic utilization. The increased activity of an enzyme which assists in ascorbate biosynthesis may be viewed as a mechanism which tends to offset decreased production of noradrenaline and subsequently of adrenaline (thereby enhancing increased c-AMP production) by Le Chatelier's principle. It could also be viewed as an example of the pattern whereby increased production of ascorbic acid resists the effect of "biochemical stress" which accompanies the uptake of the drugs. The significance of biochemical stress will be considered further in section 7.3.

5.4. Apparent inability to biosynthesize ascorbic acid

The ability of numerous mammals—such as the rat, rabbit, mouse, dog and goat—to biosynthesize ascorbic acid contrasts with the need for exogenous supply of the vitamin by other mammals such as man and the guinea pig. Following investigations employing microsomal fractions and supernatant fractions by the schools of Lehninger, King and Burns, and Chatterjee (see section 5.3) it is nowadays generally presumed that the latter group of animals is unable to biosynthesize ascorbic acid because it is unable to carry out the stages in which D-glucurono-γ-lactone and L-gulono-γ-lactone are involved in conversion to the vitamin. As a result it has been suggested that the biosynthetic deficiency is due to a "missing step" or "gene mutation" involving one or more of the following:

(a) the microsomal enzyme D-glucurono-γ-lactone reductase,

(b) L-gulono-γ-lactone oxidase, and

(c) aldonolactonase (uronolactonase).

Several classes of explanation may be advanced for the genetic absence of enzyme activities. These comprise deficiencies in the genetic material or in its expression, at either the level of transcription or translation.

At the level of the genome, the genes coding for the missing enzyme(s) might be entirely absent as the result of deletion of genetic material, or might be present but defective because of mutations which render their protein products inactive.

Even if the structural genes coding for the enzyme(s) are present, other defects might prevent their expression. Such regulator mutations might prevent transcription or translation. At the level of transcription, a defect might involve either the synthesis of hnRNA (the precursor to mRNA) or the production of messenger RNA. At the translational level, messenger might be synthesized but fail to be utilized as a template for protein synthesis.

No investigations appear to have been reported in this connection (in respect of ascorbic acid), and until the above possibilities have been thoroughly examined it is not possible to come to a definite conclusion on whether the defective formation of L-ascorbic acid in man and other animals can be attributed to missing structural gene(s).

It is desirable to draw attention to the contribution of mitochondria to the later stages of ascorbic acid biosynthesis. Indeed, Burns et al. (1956) noted that rat liver mitochondria—in contrast to guinea pig mitochondria—contributed about one quarter of the biosynthesis of ascorbic acid, as compared to the microsomal fractions.

It cannot be overemphasized that the activities of a mixture of two biological constituents is not necessarily equal to the sum of their individual contributions; rather it is the case that "deviations" may well be introduced. Thus if two constituents separately do not contribute to the biosynthesis of ascorbic acid, a mixture of the two may give rise to another factor which under proper compartmentalization will assist ascorbic acid biosynthesis. It is such possibilities that make extrapolation from in vitro to in vivo biological activities rather difficult (see also section 8.2.1).

At this stage it is worth while drawing attention to the observations of Baker *et al.* (1962). The results of their studies with healthy men revealed that when D-glucurono*lactone*-6-C^{14} was administered, about one quarter was converted to L-ascorbic acid, whereas no activity could be detected in the ascorbate derivatives isolated from the urine of subjects to whom D-glucuronic *acid*-6-C^{14} was administered. This finding contrasts with previous results *in vivo* of Burns and Evans (1956) that guinea pigs could not convert D-glucurono-lactone-6-C^{14} and L-gulonolactone-1-C^{14} to L-ascorbic acid, whereas rats did convert appreciable quantities of both compounds. It also contrasts with the conclusion that humans cannot synthesize L-ascorbic acid from D-glucuronolactone. On the basis of the established schemes (see Fig. 5.2) the conversion found by Baker *et al.* (1962) can take place only if both D-glucurono-γ-lactone-reductase and L-gulono-γ-lactone-oxidase are present in the synthesizing organ(s) of man. The finding that only a quarter of D-glucuronolactone ingested was converted to L-ascorbic acid is consistent with the possibility that the rest was hydrolysed, possibly via uronolactonase, or that the subsequent L-gulonolactone was reversibly hydrolysed via gulono-lactonase present, thereby enabling it to be shunted into the xylulose path instead of proceeding via the ascorbic acid pathway. It is desirable to establish with certainty whether human mitochondria participate in the ascorbic biosynthetic pathway and whether the difference in vitamin C requirement—often attributed to biochemical individuality—is associated with different activities of formation of uronolactonase and/or aldonolactonase. Further, since PDE hydrolyses the γ-lactone ring of ascorbate, the question arises as to the extent of the effect PDE exerts on the needs of vitamin C in human and other species. These problems will be considered also in Chapter 8.

5.5. Catabolism of L-ascorbate in animals

5.5.1. Metabolism of ascorbic acid: limitations of extrapolation from different animals to man

In Fig. 1.4 an outline was given of work on the direction of change when ascorbic acid is oxidized *in vitro*; and one can understand the attempt to extrapolate this to humans. Most of the investigations on the metabolism of ascorbic acid have been carried out on animals such as the rat and guinea pig. It is difficult to be certain as to the limits of extrapolation from such species to humans. To illustrate this point, while it has been shown that L-ascorbic acid is converted to urinary oxalate in man (Hellman and Burns, 1958), guinea pig (Burns et al., 1951) and rat (Curtin and King, 1955), other investigations carried out to demonstrate the high extent of conversion of ascorbic acid to oxalate in rat and guinea pig tissues have been unsuccessful (Chan et al., 1958; Burns et al., 1958). In vitro it was demonstrated that L-ascorbic acid is converted to L-threonic acid and oxalate (Cox et al., 1932; Herbert et al., 1933), but this pathway has not, at any rate so far, been demonstrated in man. It is apposite to emphasize that the degradation of DHA need not proceed via 2:3-diketogulonic acid but that it can be decarboxylated to give L-xylose; this pathway was demonstrated by Chan et al. (1958) in guinea pigs. Further, Kanfer et al. (1960) and Shimanozo and Mano (1961) have shown that diketogulonic acid is degraded to L-lyxonic acid and to L-xylonic acid in rat kidney.

The catabolism of ascorbate can take place via the ascorbic free radical to be followed by the oxidative pathway or by formation of free radicals in other substances. Alternatively, the ascorbate can be hydrolysed by PDE—as outlined in Chapter 3—to the delactonized form (DEL-AA) which may then follow the oxidative pathway. Further, there exists evidence that—in guinea pigs or rats—L-ascorbate, the DHA and diketogulonate are converted into glucose (e.g. Dayton et al., 1959; Rudolff et al., 1956; Chan et al., 1958) and that D-glucuronolactone (Burns et al., 1957; Eisenberg et al., 1959) and xylitol, which can be formed by reduction from both L-xylulose and D-xylulose (Touster et al., 1956; Hollman and Touster, 1957), can be converted into glycogen.

5.5.2. Oxidative path of L-ascorbate

On the basis of the results of various investigations (for numerous references, see, for example, Degkwitz, 1965; Burns, 1967) it has been concluded that the oxidation of L-ascorbate results in the production of DHA, 2:3-diketogulonic acid, oxalate, xylose, L-xylonate, L-lyxonate, xylulose and CO_2. Much of the work was carried out on rats and guinea pigs, and some of the conclusions have by inference been extrapolated to man although a number of investigations were carried out directly on human tissue extracts and on man himself. The individual quantities of the various substances formed vary within the results of a single group of researchers as well as between different groups. See Table 3.1 for variations of half-life times. It is apposite to emphasize that different paths may be followed in the oxidation of ascorbate (as shown in Fig. 1.4) and that the same product may be excreted in different outlets (as pointed out in Fig. 3.1). The probability of the route(s) followed depends on the diet, hormonal changes which can be influenced by circumstances and by intake of drugs. It is therefore not surprising that the extent of metabolism of ascorbate leading to expired CO_2 is in dispute. Burns (1967) claims categorically that "no conversion of L-ascorbic acid-1-^{14}C to respiratory CO_2 was detected in man". Hellman and Burns (1958) found less than 5.0% of administered ^{14}C-L-ascorbic acid in humans in contrast with the much higher percentages found in guinea pigs and in rats (Burns et al., 1951). Abt et al. (1963) found an average of 18 to 21% of the ingested ascorbate as expired CO_2, and Atkins et al. (1964) found between 44 and 57%. Such wide differences may in part be attributed to biochemical individuality; they also illustrate the difficulties in making unequivocal statements as to ascorbate involvement and performance in humans.

It is pertinent to note the observations of Chatterjee et al. (1975) who concluded that feeding of animals on cereal diet and ascorbic acid results in a high proportion of DHA in blood and other tissues. Such a result suggests blockage of the mechanism by which ascorbic acid is regenerated, resulting in DHA being broken down to 2:3-diketogluconic acid and its products.

5.6. Calcium metabolism

5.6.1. Calcium and ascorbate blood levels

Increased levels of ascorbate in blood should result in decreased ionized Ca levels, as Ca complexes with ascorbate (see section 1.2.7).

The trend for blood clotting depends inter alia on the Ca levels in blood. There is evidence that, in vitro, ascorbated blood clots a little more slowly than normal blood. However, the overall pattern appears more complex since there is some evidence, discussed below, that increased ascorbate intake can increase mobilization of freshly deposited Ca in bone and this would tend to oppose decreased Ca levels.

5.6.2. Bone metabolism

Bone formation involves orderly deposition of Ca salts within the matrix of collagen. Ascorbate is known to be essential to the biosynthesis of collagen (for extensive reviews see Barnes and Kodicek, 1972). However, it is not certain to what extent ascorbate is directly involved in Ca deposition in bone. It is relevant that the introduction of high concentrations of ascorbate (at levels of 10 mg/100 g of body weight) to diets of male chicks, 6 days after administration of [45]Ca, resulted in increased blood levels of the isotope within 4 to 8 hours of the introduction of the ascorbate, but that after 24 hours this effect was lost and eventually normal levels were attained (Thornton, 1968). As plasma acid phosphatase activity was elevated following ascorbate injection and since total plasma Ca was depressed by the ascorbate, this indicates that the effect on bone was indirect. Since mobilization of bone salt is generally considered to be controlled by a parathyroid hormone (PTH) (Arnaud *et al.*, 1967) and since decrease in soluble ionic calcium levels results in secretion of this hormone the effect could be considered to be an example of hormone control. Thornton (1970) considers that this is not the case. However, there is now a considerable body of evidence which indicates that the bone-mobilization effect of PTH is mediated by c-AMP (for references, see Robison *et al.*, 1971). Now, since c-AMP levels are likely to be raised as a result of ascorbate competition with c-AMP for the active sites in PDE (see section 4.9.2) a relationship between increased ascorbate levels and Ca metabolism is indicated. Such an effect would be counteracted by the decreased levels of soluble ionic Ca, thereby tending to act as a feed-back mechanism.

The pattern of preferential mobilization of recently deposited [45]Ca from bone is interesting, but it does not necessarily signify destruction of bone-tissue as inferred by Thornton. Freshly precipitated material is usually more soluble than older crystals, because thermodynamic equilibrium is attained rather slowly (for explanations, see Lewin, 1960, 1974a). The [45]Ca used was comparatively freshly precipitated, and thus its mobilization followed the principle "last in, first out". It is relevant that the bone tissue constituents are in dynamic equilibrium with the surrounding fluids. The [45]Ca mobilization—in contrast with the reduced overall Ca levels in the plasma—does not necessarily indicate increased bone metabolism leading to bone destruction, but rather implies that there is preferential exchange of freshly deposited material between bone tissue and the surroundings. The possible significance of this phenomenon is that over-calcification of tissues, generally of more recent origin than normal bone growth, can be reversed as a result of the increased reversible activity exhibited on increased intake of ascorbate. In this sense increased intake of ascorbate may assist "normal" processes, physiologically controlled, thereby reducing excessive calcification. This aspect deserves a thorough investigation which should encompass the problem of how far the significance of results obtained on chicks can be extrapolated to humans, and to what extent the drinking of hard water influences the results.

Chapter 6

Biological transport and storage, and steady state levels

6.1. Energy and transport aspects

Biological transport activities are conveniently divided into those of ordinary transport and those of active transport; ordinary transport takes place by spontaneous diffusion, whereas active transport is motivated and financed by energy supply. Diffusion of solutes from higher concentrations into lower ones is motivated by a decrease in free energy; this driving force is negated when the two concentrations are equal. Movement of solutes from lower concentrations into higher concentrations is opposed by diffusion and can take place only when the energy required for the process is donated by an associated reaction, and is normally termed active transport. The pumping of blood by the heart is an example of a mechanically motivated active transport; it can enforce transport of water across semipermeable membranes from media where it is dilute into media where it is concentrated, against the osmotic pressure. The energy required for the process is supplied by the muscles which in turn obtain it from a series of suitably sequenced energy donor reactions. Compartmentalization is always utilized by biological systems in concentrating solutes, and the membranes employed often are semipermeable. Further, the mechanisms utilized for active transport vary with the particular tissues and the surrounding medium.

From perusal of Table 4.1 it will be appreciated that the concentration of ascorbate in the various listed tissues is many times that present in blood (where the "normal" range may vary from approximately 0.8 to 2.0 mg per 100 mls plasma (Friedman *et al.,* 1940). Since the ascorbate in food finds its way, after absorption, into the blood, whence it is transported elsewhere, it follows that

118

some active transport must be responsible for the greater ascorbate concentrations in the other tissues.

Considerable information is available concerning active transport in general, but relatively little is known concerning that of ascorbate, as will be appreciated from the following.

The characteristics of active transport processes have been shown to involve

(i) Energy-donating sources;
(ii) transportee specificity;
(iii) dependence of the rate of transport on the concentration of the transportee, the kinetics of the rate being similar to those of enzyme kinetics;
(iv) directional specificity; and
(v) selective poisoning.

It is also generally recognized that active transport mechanisms involve their respective specific carrier proteins and specific energy-transfer proteins.

Ascorbate is known to be transported partly unattached—e.g. from blood, via the porous blood vessel walls into the lymph—and partly bound (e.g. Sumerwell and Sealocki, 1952; Roe and Itscoitz, 1963; Nichelmann *et al.*, 1966), but the type of binding has not been established. It has also been established that ascorbate penetrates erythrocyte membranes very slowly in comparison with the oxidized form, DHA (e.g. Martin, 1961; Hughes and Maton, 1968). Transport is accomplished by oxidizing the ascorbate to DHA which after penetrating into the cell is reduced to ascorbate by reduced gluta-thione. Thus the transport of ascorbate into the erythrocyte involves a cycle comprising at least two different processes (accompanied by energy financing reactions).

The complexity of and the differences between ascorbate uptake by different tissues may be appreciated from the following.

Sherry and Ralli (1948) reported that both *in vitro* and *in vivo* insulin caused a transfer of ascorbate into leucocytes but not into erythrocytes. Hughes and Maton (1968) reported that the uptake of ascorbate by erythrocytes did not appear to be influenced by enzyme inhibition. McIlwain *et al.* (1956) suggested that ascorbate uptake in brain is energy assisted. Sharma *et al.* (1963) concluded that the uptake of ascorbate in brain cortex and adrenal cortex of guinea pigs is an energy-dependent process, and that ouabain and 2:4-dinitrophenol suppress ascorbate uptake into brain cortex slices; also, ACTH was found to inhibit uptake of ascorbate in adrenal cortex but not in brain cortex slices; they suggested that ACTH inhibits the uptake of ascorbate in the adrenal cortex through the steroids produced in its presence. Mann and Newton (1974) found that D-glucose, D-mannose, D-xylose, D-galactose, and D-arabinose (in this order) strongly inhibit the uptake of DHA by erythrocytes; but DHA transport is facilitated by Cu ions. Little is known of the molecular mechanism of active transport of ascorbate into leucocytes and other tissues and of the mechanisms of release of the ascorbate when required. Nevertheless, it is apposite to consider stereochemically and energetically admissible mechanisms by which these processes may be accomplished.

First let us consider the energy requirements in active processes involving the ascorbate transport against a concentration gradient. The free energy required (ΔG) to transport a neutral molecule from a lower concentration (C_l) to a higher concentration (C_h) is given by the relation:

$$\Delta G = 2.303 \, RT\{\log_{10}(C_h/C_l)\} \text{ calories per mole}, \qquad (6.1)$$

where R is the gas constant and T is the absolute temperature.

The variation of ΔG with the concentration ratio at 37°C has been computed, and the data are presented in Table 6.1.

Table 6.1. Variation of the free energy required for active transport with concentration ratio

(C_h/C_l)	10	20	30	40	50	60	70	80	90	100
ΔG(kcal per mole)	1.43	1.86	2.11	2.29	2.43	2.54	2.64	2.72	2.74	2.86

It will be appreciated that the free energy required per mole transported increases linearly (by 1.43 kcal) for every tenfold increase in concentration ratio.

The transport of an ion against its ionic concentration gradient involves more work than that required for a neutral molecule. However, it can be computed that the total free energy required (that is to effect transport against the combined concentration gradients) runs parallel to that given in Table 6.1. The precise values are difficult to compute unless the overall ionic strengths in the two separated media, the nature of any accompanying cation as well as the nature of the protein-carrier and the respective availability of water, are known. However, it may be assumed that in the normal physiological ranges (and when the transport of the ascorbate is accompanied either by its own counterion or by an oppositely directed transport of other anionic species) the corresponding free energies required will not exceed twice those given in Table 6.1. Thus the approximate energy requirements will be no higher than 3 kcal for a tenfold and 6 kcal for a hundredfold concentration ratio.

Such energy requirements are amply satisfied by energy-donor processes, e.g.

$$\text{ATP} \xrightarrow{\text{Hydrolysis}} \text{ADP} + \text{Pi} \quad \Delta G^{\circ} = -7.3 \text{ kcal/mole}$$

$$\text{Glucose} \xrightarrow{\text{Glycolysis}} 2 \text{ Lactate} \quad \Delta G^{\circ} = -47 \text{ kcal/mole}$$

The oxidation of ascorbate to DHA can be linked to the reduction of a number of cytochromes (or other suitable substances) which have higher positive redox emf values at the physiological concentrations. A number of cytochromes can be chosen of which the standard redox reduction emfs should be more positive than that of E_o (oxidation) for AA → DHA. Their E_o values (for reduction) range from +0.29 to +0.12 (see Table 2.2). The E_o (oxidation) of AA → DHA is −0.058. In illustration we can choose cytochrome c with E_o (reduction) = +0.25; the E_o of the combination is then c. +0.19. The resulting free energy change is

$$\Delta G^{\circ} = -nFE_o = \frac{-2 \times 96,500 \times 0.19}{4.185 \times 1000} = -8.76 \text{ kcal/mole}$$

This value is much higher than those given in Table 6.1 and illustrates the ability of the oxidation of ascorbate to finance the energy requirements of its own active transport as DHA across the membrane of the erythrocyte. It may therefore be that the method of transport of ascorbate into erythrocytes has been selected by evolution to enable passage through permeable lipid membranes as well as to provide simultaneously the necessary energy for the first stage of the transport.

6.2. Means of transport

6.2.1. Transport media

Ascorbate is transported from the plasma to the non-motile erythrocytes and by the motile leucocytes to other tissues. The mechanism has probably evolved on the basis of efficiency. The threshold urinary excretion range is around 1.4 to 1.8 mg per 100 ml of glomerular fluid. In the absence of leucocytes capable of extracting ascorbate from the plasma to a c. forty- to fifty-fold concentration, the loss via the glomeruli could be costly.

6.2.2. Blood-lymph transporting activities

The ascorbate in the blood is propelled into the lymph via the pores in the membranes of the walls of the blood vessels. Unattached ascorbate is a comparatively small molecule which can pass readily with the fluid through the pores into the lymphatic spaces; it can also be carried by the leucocytes as they penetrate into the intercellular spaces of the blood vessel walls. In this manner ascorbate moves out from the blood into the lymph spaces at the arterial end and re-enters the vascular system at the venous end.

6.2.3. Chemotaxis

Chemotaxis appears to play a role in the direction of ascorbate transport by the leucocytes. Leucocytes are known to migrate towards wound-areas and infarcted myocardia. Thus, Hume *et al.* (1972) observed that leucocytes move towards infarcted myocardia and deposit ascorbate there. This movement is probably chemotactic and is triggered by the release of histamine from local mast cells. Preliminary experiments I have carried out indicate that leucocytes migrate preferentially towards areas having higher histamine concentrations.

6.2.4. Mega ascorbate intake and tissue uptake

It has been claimed by some writers that uptake of ascorbate from administration of over c. 100 mg daily results in "tissue saturation", the inference being that higher intakes are simply wasted, because of the glomerular threshhold limit of c. 1.4 to 1.9 mg ascorbate per 100 ml of the glomerular fluid. This "saturation" argument is untenable for several reasons given below, and should be discarded.

Variation in the maximum concentration values of ascorbate in plasma. It cannot be over-emphasized that the existence of a renal threshold (between 1.1 and 1.9 mg per 100 ml of plasma; see for example Kyhos *et al.*, 1945) does *not* exclude temporary steady state levels with significantly higher ascorbate concentration. The steady state levels depend on the rate of input of the ascorbate and the rate of its removal. The rate of removal via the renal system is limited by the capacity of the glomeruli for filtration. Sufficiently rapid "topping up" of ascorbate in the plasma can therefore over-compensate for the rate of loss via the urine and thus raise the steady state levels. Indeed, the so-called "saturated state" of vitamin C in the plasma is by no means a saturated state, nor is it a fixed steady state with a limited ascorbate concentration level. The upper limit has been found to vary from 1.4 mg to almost 4 mg per 100 ml of plasma depending on the quantity of ascorbate/ascorbic acid ingested, and on the frequency of ingestion (see section 7.7.2.3 and Fig. 7.2).

Distinction between "saturated state" and "steady state". The raised levels of vitamin C in the plasma, following greatly increased intakes of the vitamin, do *not* represent a *saturated state* the level of which is controlled by the renal threshold, but rather *steady states* which result from dynamic interchange of the ascorbate between plasma, lymph and tissues, and a renal threshold which varies widely between 1.1 and 1.9 mg per 100 ml of plasma (e.g. Kyhos *et al.,* 1945). Two factors are important in controlling the level of ascorbic acid:

(a) Increasing absorption of the vitamin by the tissues due to special pumping mechanism from the lymph and from the plasma into particular cells/tissues where raised levels of activity and storage of the vitamin persist; and

(b) Increasing excretion due to a renal threshold which limits rises in the plasma level of the vitamin.

The difference between the following situations should assist clarification:

Uptake limited by concentration gradients

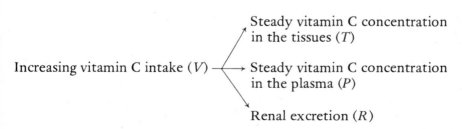

Increasing vitamin C intake (V)

Steady vitamin C concentration in the tissues (T)

Steady vitamin C concentration in the plasma (P)

Renal excretion (R)

$V = R + T + P$ when V *increases to* V', $V' = R' + T + P$ where $V - V$
$= R' - R$.

Uptake enhanced by pumping mechanisms (which overcome
concentration gradients)

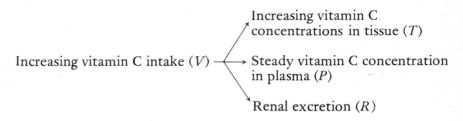

Increasing vitamin C intake (*V*)

Increasing vitamin C
concentrations in tissue (*T*)

Steady vitamin C concentration
in plasma (*P*)

Renal excretion (*R*)

$V = R + T + P$. When V increases to V', T and R and P increases
to T', R' and P' respectively, T' and R' can increase greatly; the rise in
$P \rightarrow P'$ consequently lags well behind.

The factors which tend to restrict the increase in value of P within
comparatively small steady state ranges of 1.4 to 3 mg/100 ml plasma
are:

(i) the difference of {(hydrostatic pressure) − (osmotic pressure)} in the blood, and the permeability of the walls of the
capillary to the small molecule of the vitamin. Here there is
apparently no threshold.

(ii) Uptake by the leucocytes and other tissues which possess
powerful pumping mechanisms in the active transport of the
vitamin, thus

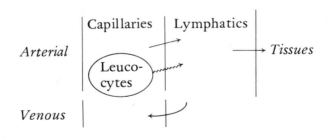

It is apposite to draw attention to the significance of the determinations of vitamin C in blood; these are usually carried out on venous
blood. This blood contains the ascorbate left after delivery to the
various tissues. Hence the *venous* vitamin C concentration should be
lower than the *arterial* concentration. Further, any determinations of

blood ascorbate subsequent to the passage through the kidney are bound to be lower than in the arterial system prior to filtration in the glomeruli.

Increasing vitamin C concentrations in the plasma enable higher intake by the tissues, according to equation 6.1. For a given available energy in a particular active transport, the greater the C_{plasma} (i.e. C_l), the higher is the value of C_h in the tissues. These conclusions are in accord with the experimental findings of Kübler and Gehler (1970) who showed that increased ingestion of vitamin C over the range of 1.5 to 12 g daily results in increasing absorption of the vitamin, over the percentage ratio of (absorbed/ingested) ascorbate decrease. See also Fig. 7.2.

6.3. Storage and release mechanisms

A number of stereochemically and energetically admissible mechanisms can be outlined for storage and release:

The *upkeep* of high concentrations of ascorbate can be ensured by the presence of high concentrations of chemical groups which can combine with it, e.g. guanidinium group of arginine (see also section 1.2.8.2) and hydroxyl groups on adjacent carbon atoms (see section 1.2.8.3) such as in adrenaline or tartrates. Thereby a lower concentration of *free* ascorbate is enforced within the particular cell or tissue which may equal the concentration of free ascorbate in the surrounding fluid.

Stored/bound ascorbate can be released from its bound state (see below).* In the erythrocyte this would be followed by oxidation to DHA which can then penetrate the cell membrane and hence escape to the plasma, followed by reduction to ascorbate. However, the process of oxidation to DHA and reduction to ascorbate, while followed in erythrocytes, need not be postulated in leucocytes where the permeability of the membrane may well increase with change in shape.

On the basis of the use of correctly proportioned space filling molecular models and energy considerations it is possible to advance stereochemically and energetically *admissible* mechanisms, as are given below.

---

* The guanidinium cation should associate more readily with double-negatively charged oxyanion than with single negatively charged analogues. Hence, $SO_4^=$ or $HPO_4^=$ should be able to dislodge ascorbate from its association with guanidinium.

*Ascorbate binding to guanidinium (arginine) group or to an ε-ammonium group of a protein**

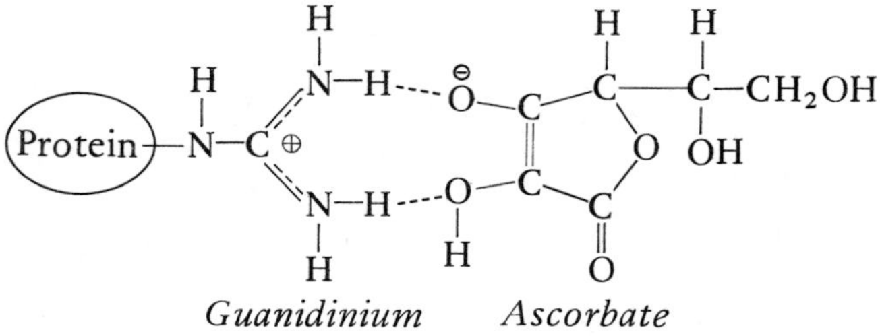

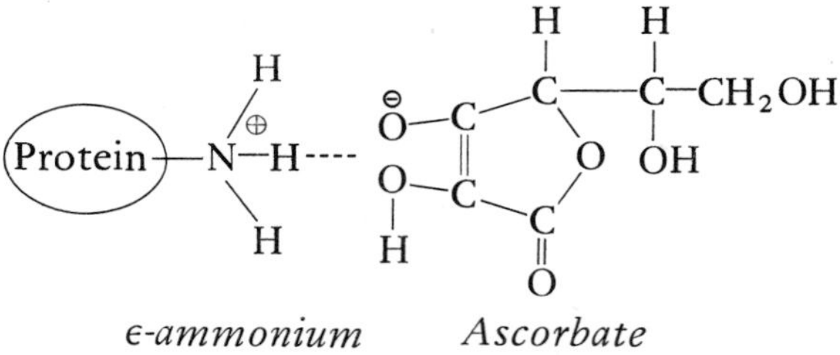

Guanidinium   Ascorbate

ε-ammonium   Ascorbate

Liberation from such linkage can be achieved by attachment of a carboxylate group with a lower pK value, or a phosphate (double negatively charged), or a sulphate ion, thus

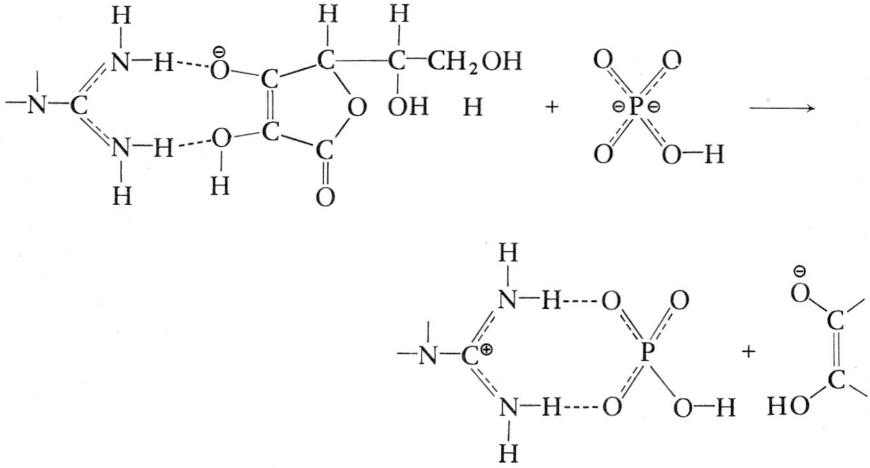

---

* It can readily be computed that the guanidinium ascorbate linkage is stronger than the ammonium ascorbate linkage (2H... bonds as compared to an equivalent of one H... bond).

Ascorbate binding to a group with two hydroxyl groups on neighbouring carbons

This binding is illustrated in Fig. 1.7.

Liberation of the ascorbate from its bound state can be attained by its attachment to a doubly charged cation, thus

Ascorbate

Association of DHA with N—H groups of a random coil, thus

Liberation of the ascorbate accompanies the formation of an α-helix from the random coil, as a result of H... bonding between the >NH groups and the >CO groups.

In the case of polypeptides possessing appropriately sited hydrophobic groups, adherence can tilt the balance towards the helix form. Hence, a rise in interfacial tension (see sections 1.2.6, 2.4.2 and 2.4.3) can tilt the balance towards the helix, thereby displacing the DHA. A sufficient lowering of the interfacial tension can tilt the balance towards the random coil thereby enabling formation of polypeptide ascorbate linkage.

Part III

Medical aspects of high intake of vitamin C, genetic aspects and future developments

Chapter 7

Medical potential of high intake of vitamin C

7.1. Controversial aspects and their resolution

There are many reports in the literature enumerating medical benefits of high intake of ascorbic acid; there are also statements by several established researchers that they have failed to confirm such claims. Often a confusing situation is encountered where ascorbic acid "believers" and "non-believers" consider that the other side is prejudiced. The "non-believers" further consider that a scientifically valid case has not been presented either theoretically or experimentally in favour of mega vitamin C therapy or prophylaxis, and that dangers exist in mega administration which outweigh any possible therapeutic/prophylactic potential. However, the argument that there is no theoretical basis for the concept that mega intake of vitamin C is beneficial is no longer tenable because of the evidence marshalled and particularly because of the pattern advanced here for the link between ascorbate levels and cyclic nucleotide levels (or PDE inhibition) and because of the potential of AFR to promote anti-viral and other beneficial activities. Discrepancies between the results of different schools of investigators and between those of individuals in the same group could be due to different proportions of absorption of the administered vitamin. From what has been outlined previously it is reasonable to suggest that discrepancies between positive and negative results originate in different extents of oxidative degradation of the vitamin when following different methods of intake, and in varying hydrolytic deactivation abilities possessed by different individuals and due to different diets.

In Chapter 4 were outlined several aspects of the physiological effects of AA in respect of PDE inhibition and thereby on c-AMP and c-GMP levels, and their potential to inhibit/retard some malfunctions. It is known that normal functioning of physiological

131

activities requires particular hormone-balance activities and controls mediated via the activities of the cyclic nucleotides. Factors which affect the normal levels of these nucleotides must therefore also affect normal physiological activities. We have therefore a basis on which to examine these aspects further and collate them within the conceptual framework which covers the medical potential of mega vitamin C intake and which encompasses the effects of different methods of administration and assay of the vitamin and different responses caused by variations in biochemical individuality.

There are two major approaches which we can employ to draw the pattern which should resolve the controversy concerning the usefulness of mega intake of vitamin C. One is first to classify the available information (and contradictory aspects) and then ask ourselves how far the impact of ascorbate on cyclic nucleotide concentration levels can be used to explain the contradictions. The second is to determine how far biologically active vitamin C concentrations in the tissues are influenced by mega intake of AA and to what extent the effect on cyclic nucleotide concentration levels can in turn express itself prophylactically/therapeutically in physiological patterns associated with body malfunctions; further, to ascertain any resultant undesirable side effects and any biochemical variations which can be encountered in different individuals.

Whatever approach is employed in assessing the medical potential of AA it is necessary to consider to what extent individual malfunctions are caused by foreign agencies which can be deactivated by AFR and/or by irregularities in the cyclic nucleotide physiological pattern, and how much by other irregularities which may or may not be open to correction by higher AA levels. In the process we have also to consider the meaning of a number of terms commonly used in the literature such as biochemical stress, the common cold, and other malfunctions. The first approach has been exercised to some extent in the preceding chapters. Greater emphasis will now be afforded to developing and applying the second approach within the conceptual framework.

7.2. Methodology of administration and associated deactivation of vitamin C

7.2.1. Deactivation and methodology

Ascorbic acid/ascorbate may be administered in several ways, e.g. intravenous injection, oral infeed, drip-feed or subcutaneous injection; the last two are rarely used. However, unless optimal conditions are enforced, the administration of a quantity of the vitamin may well result in only a fractional uptake resulting from oxidative degradation prior to absorption via the alimentary system, and from hydrolysis of the lactone structure.

7.2.2. Methodology

The most suitable form in which the vitamin should be offered to the human body depends on its site of entry.

Intravenous injection: The vitamin should obviously be offered in aqueous, physiologically acceptable, solution as ascorbate. The solution should be anaerobic* and should contain physiologically acceptable chelating agents, such as amino acids or citrate,* so as to retard pre-administration aerobic oxidation which is catalysed by dissolved traces of copper and iron.

The ascorbate is best prepared from the acid form. The solid acid form can be kept stable for years if stored in the dark under nitrogen and at temperatures below $c.$ 20–30°C. The computed quantity of the acid can then be neutralized with an equivalent amount of NaOH, or with bicarbonate. The following precautions are essential if the deactivation of the vitamin is to be reduced to a minimum.

  (i) Solution preparation must take place in very subdued lighting; the preparation vessel and the stored sample and transfers must be shielded from light. Anaerobic conditions should be enforced.
  (ii) The aqueous medium should contain the biologically suitable chelating agent *before* dissolving the vitamin.
  (iii) Keeping the solution frozen at −70°C assists in retardation of deactivation—as judged by optical absorbance and by PDE hydrolysis.

Under such conditions the solutions usually retain their biological activities for two to three weeks, or longer.

Oral administration: Oral intake can be achieved in various ways such as swallowing of tablets or capsules with water,† the dissolving of vitamin C powder in a suitable aqueous solution, chewing of the

---

* Lamden and Kunin (1970) concluded that ascorbate assists decomposition of citrate (when the citrate is chelated to Cu^{++}) when the solution is shaken with air, and in presence of background lighting; but that gassing with nitrogen offsets this catalysis. Amino acids chelate Cu^{++} or Fe^{++} far more effectively than citrates.

† Warm aqueous fluids enhance opening of the pyloric sphincter thereby favouring quicker absorption of the vitamin.

tablets or the use of slow-release capsules. Each of these procedures has its own vitamin deactivating pitfalls. Three stages exist where vitamin C deactivation is likely to occur in oral administration, namely in the preparatory stage prior to swallowing, in the passage through the duodenum, and subsequently in transport along the intestines.

Vitamin C is comparatively quickly deactivated when dissolved in tap water; as much as 50% can be deactivated within two to four hours, because the neutral pH of the tap water favours the formation of the ascorbate anion which is catalytically oxidized by the air present via the traces of iron and copper normally found in water. Dissolving the ascorbic acid in orange juice or grapefruit juice or in amino acid solutions retards deactivation as the iron and copper are greatly complexed with the citric acid/citrate present in the fruit juice or with the amino acids. However, this procedure has so far not been universally employed.

Effervescent vitamin C tablets—containing sodium bicarbonate—possess an advantage in that the CO_2 emerging expels the air present in the solution and thus reduces deactivation. However, the sodium content of the tablets would be unacceptable to individuals who have to restrict their sodium intake.

In the duodenum, the pH of the food being digested tends to be neutral or alkaline. This condition and the comparatively high oxygen content in the duodenum favour oxidation of the vitamin to DHA which is liable to rapid oxidative degradation. Different diets affect the degree of neutrality of the contents of the duodenum as well as its oxygen content to different extents.* This could result in the vitamin C orally administered being decimated in the duodenum in some individuals, whereas in others the loss would be minimal.

The misfortunes of the vitamin are not restricted to the duodenum. On entry into the intestine it encounters a new enemy in the form of PDE. The bacterial flora[†] flourish and disintegrate in the intestines, and the bacterial PDE is bound to be shed with their debris into the digested food containing the ascorbate which escaped execution in the duodenum. The lactone structure of the vitamin now undergoes a hydrolysis onslaught at the fairly neutral pH values in the intestine. Mg^{++} (or Co^{++}, or Zn^{++}, Mn^{++}) are essential for

---

* Diets containing protein exert a protective influence on ascorbate, because the resultant peptides and amino acids effectively chelate cations such as those of copper, iron and magnesium.

† E. coli have been shown to be a source of PDE (e.g. Brana and Chytil, 1966; Monard *et al.*, 1969).

PDE activity. It can therefore reasonably be expected that in some individuals in whom the ionic magnesium content is favourable to the activity of phosphodiesterase (e.g. in protein-free and chelating-free media), hydrolytic rupture of the lactone ring of the vitamin would be pronounced, thereby leading to further decimation of any ascorbate that has escaped from the duodenum.

The timing of oral ingestion of the mega ascorbic dose varies. Some individuals take their AA dose with protein-free meals. The digested meal is an ideal nutrient for the bacterial flora, and the longer the ascorbate—when taken in a chelation-free medium—is in contact with the bacterial flora, the greater is the probability of the PDE from decomposed bacteria deactivating the vitamin by hydrolytic action. In contrast ascorbate taken orally between meals is less likely to encounter a mass of bacterial flora, and if taken with amino acids or citrates the associated chelating activity for divalent cations should retard PDE activity.

We thus have a basis for differentiation in respect of vitamin C absorption in terms of different times of intake, diets and individuals. An intake of 1 g of vitamin C in some individuals may result in only a few milligrams being available for absorption while in others a much greater proportion would be absorbed. Only when the research projects on mega vitamin C medical uses take cognizance of these variables will it be possible to say with certainty whether any negative results noted can be ascribed to non-absorption of the administered vitamin, or to its non-effectiveness. A measure of the extent of absorption could be arrived at by determining any increase in vitamin C content in the blood and collating this with the clinical effects noted. However, all vitamin C assays reported in the literature have relied on the reducing power of ascorbate (e.g. on the 2:6-dichlorophenolindophenol titre), or assay optical absorbance, of phenylhydrazone products of DHA and 2:3 dibetagulonic acid. As pointed out in Chapter 3, these methods determine the sum-total of {[AA] + [Del-A]} but the current procedures have not been devised with the object of differentiating between the biologically active [AA] and the biologically inactive [Del-A]. Although it is probable that an increase in the dichlorophenolindophenol titre would, under otherwise identical conditions, reflect an increase in AA concentration, this presumes absence of variation in PDE activity. A valid vitamin assay requires recognition of the potential of PDE to hydrolyse the lactone structure of ascorbate; and care must be taken on the lines suggested in Chapter 3 to assess its activity. It cannot be over-emphasized that, currently, insufficient information is available regarding the overall potential of PDE to hydrolyse AA. Thus, it is not known yet whether AA bound to particular proteins resists hydrolysis by PDE. We are not yet in a position to answer the question of whether or how far Del-A can be reformed into AA under physiological conditions. Until precise answers to these questions are obtained and until the variations in different individuals are delineated, correspondingly wide areas of uncertainty will remain (see also sections 8.3 and 9.3).

Nevertheless, in view of the outlined potential of ascorbate to enhance numerous biological activities and to oppose body malfunctioning directly and indirectly, the variations in medical benefits noted following mega *administration* of AA can be understood within the conceptual framework that high absorption (as compared to ingestion) of vitamin C is beneficial to resistance to malfunction and that variations occur because of different extents of deactivation of the vitamin prior to administration or thereafter (see also section 8.3).

7.3. Vitamin C utilization in relation to biological activities

Vitamin C utilization depends on the level of activity in which the constituents of the ascorbic system (AA, AFR, DHA) are involved, and the extent to which the vitamin is degraded or deactivated by irreversible oxidations and delactonization. The greater the rate of redox utilization and of PDE activity, the greater is likely to be the loss to be replenished. In general the greater the degree of "biochemical stress" to which individuals are subject, the greater are the associated daily needs.

"Biochemical stress" embodies a number of various stresses the resultant effects of which are increased vitamin C requirements; if these are not met, certain tissues will begin to malfunction. The subsequent inability of the human system as a whole to cope with the malfunctioning results eventually in symptoms associated with particular illnesses. The symptoms used as the criteria of vitamin C deficiency that have been adopted by the Establishment of the medical profession are those of scurvy. The daily dose required to inhibit scurvy—often termed the Recommended Daily Allowance (RDA)—is given by various medical authorities as between 10 to 125 mg daily. However, scurvy is a clinical manifestation of prolonged and extreme vitamin C deficiency. Long before the symptoms appear, subclinical deficiency of the vitamin persists in certain tissues of particular individuals, and this situation can last for some time during which the individuals' activities are increasingly below par.

Assessment of the level of ascorbate that is needed must depend on consideration of the various ways in which administration of ascorbate has been shown to be effective as well as those in which its potential has received some or no assessment. In this connection it is necessary to realize that difficulties in interpretation are caused if no differentiation is made between the following three classes of ascorbate involvement:

(i) Conditions which give rise to ascorbate deficiency;

(ii) malfunctioning caused by ascorbate deficiency, and

(iii) malfunctions which are not directly caused by ascorbate deficiency, but which can nevertheless be rectified by high concentration levels of ascorbate in the malfunctioning system (e.g. inhibition of over-activity of PDE resulting from biochemical stress, and the detoxifying action of high concentrations of AA on nitroamines).

It is not always easy to disentangle these effects, but efforts will nevertheless be made to achieve differentiation wherever possible.

7.4. Reasons for mega vitamin C administration

7.4.1. General considerations

The daily dose of ascorbate intake is dictated by the need to maintain an ascorbate reservoir in the body at a level which can readily meet the demands made upon it. The demands under "normal" conditions and those when the body is exposed to attack differ considerably. The dose required to meet normal conditions (N)—i.e. the prophylactic dose—should be lower than that required when the body is under attack (A) because physiological activities are at a correspondingly lower level in the former. The respective values of A and of N can differ multifold with the individual for the following reasons:

Ability to biosynthesize ascorbate. Some individuals should be capable of biosynthesizing ascorbate (see Chapter 8) to greater extent than others. Let the quantity required daily be d g, then

$$d = x + n$$

where x = exogenous intake, and n = endogenous production, i.e. biosynthesis. n is likely to vary with the individual's diet, as it is known that variations in diet of a number of animals can affect ascorbate biosynthesis multifold (e.g. Chatterjee *et al.*, 1975).

The daily dose. The daily exogenous ascorbate requirement ($= d - n$), which equals A or N depending on the conditions can vary enormously from, say, 50 to 5000 mg because of biochemical individuality (see section 8.3). Individuals normally not subject to mental stresses such as harrassment, worry, fear, excitement and the rat-race, should need far less ascorbate than those subject to the full rigours of modern technological/administrative life.

The quantity x is not likely to be the quantity taken up orally (the procedure by which most individuals take additional ascorbic acid) but must rather be a significantly lower value as a result of the oxidation of AA to DHA (e.g. prior to swallowing, and in the duodenum) which is rapidly degraded, and of hydrolytic deactivation by PDE present in the intestine following bacterial decomposition. The bacterial flora present in the intestine vary with the individual and the individual's diet. Bacterial decomposition and release of PDE depend on several factors such as the diet; the timing of the ingestion of ascorbic acid intake in relation to the intake of the main meal is important since the higher AA intake favours development of anaerobic bacteria.*

The eating habits of different individuals can vary considerably, and thus the proportion of the vitamin saved from deactivation varies accordingly. Having entered the blood stream the ascorbate is probably protected from oxidative degradation by association with serum proteins (preliminary experimental work I have carried out suggests that ascorbate oxidation is lowered in the presence of serum proteins) and probably from hydrolytic deactivation because of the relative absence of PDE. The overall field of biochemical individuality is considered in Chapter 8. However, it is worth while noting here that the variation is ascorbate requirements can be computed to extend about five-hundred-fold for c. 80% inhibition of overactivity of PDE, and even more for 90% inhibition.

7.4.2. Energy supply efficiency

Increased extent of physiological activity requires correspondingly more energy. This requirement can be met by increased efficiency in the process of making energy available. ATP is one of the major energy reservoirs/suppliers in biological organizations, since its breakdown to ADP or AMP releases considerable energy in forms which are linked in numerous reactions. The production of ATP in the

---

* Ascorbic acid intake should favour anaerobic bacteria at the expense of aerobic bacteria. This effect can be computed theoretically; it was considered to be the cause of gastrointestinal discomforts experienced by some individuals undergoing mega vitamin C administration (Regnier, 1968).

mitochondria requires energy transport and infeed of chemical energy made available by anaerobic and/or aerobic reactions. Ascorbate can be seen readily to assist in both formation of ATP and its breakdown. The supply of the chemical energy required for formation of ATP can be mediated by AFR—which would explain the significance of ascorbic acid oxidase (see section 2.3.2.2). Also aerobic mechanisms are more efficient than anaerobic in production of ATP. Thus glycolysis and aerobic mechanisms provide respectively 33 and 50% efficiencies in production of ATP. It is relevant therefore that high concentrations of ascorbate in incubation media result in depressed lactic acid production and increased oxygen uptake by polymorphic leucocytes; this indicates that increased ascorbate levels enhance improved efficiency in the availability of energy by favouring the more efficient aerobic processes.*

7.5. Potential *in vivo* anti-viral defence mechanisms

There are several individual contributions by ascorbate— particularly under aerated conditions—to anti-viral defence activities, some of which have been referred to previously. It is apposite to gather them in one section, as their collective effect is of considerable significance in various malaises.

Several investigators make the point directly or by implication (e.g. Walker, Bynoe and Tyrrell, 1967) that *in vitro*, ascorbate does not affect most of the viruses known to cause havoc in the common cold or in influenza. The inference generally drawn is that if ascorbate does not exhibit anti-viral effects *in vitro* there is no particular reason why it should do so *in vivo*. It is therefore desirable to stress that ascorbate can act both directly and indirectly in assisting anti-viral defence activities, thus:

Formation of AFR radicals. These assist more rapid biosynthesis of γ-globulins (see section 4.4.2) and other normal physiological activities. AFR has also been implicated in *in vitro* experiments in deactivation of several viruses and phages. Thus Murata *et al.* (1972, 1972a, b) and Murata and Kitagawa (1973) found that a number of double stranded DNA phages and RNA phages are inactivated by ascorbate when air is bubbled and oxidizing agents or transition

---

* The process ATP → ADP + Pi is accompanied by release of energy. von Euler and Klussman (1934) reported that ascorbate accelerates the hydrolytic formation of free phosphate. By increasing both the efficiency of ATP biosynthesis and the formation of free phosphate, increased ascorbate levels in the tissues should assist a more rapid energy turnover, which factor is of importance for combating biochemical stress.

metal ions are present. On the other hand bubbling of nitrogen gas, the use of reducing agents and of free radical scavengers, prevented the inactivation. The results indicated that the inactivating effect of ascorbate was oxygen dependent giving rise to the free radicals during the oxidation.*

Inhibition of catalase activity which affects results in *in-vivo* accumulation of small concentrations of H_2O_2 sufficiently lethal to the highly sensitive virulent viruses (see section 2.3.3) while hardly affecting normal tissues, and

Enhancement of biosynthesis of interferon potentiated by higher c-AMP levels which are enhanced by the increased ascorbate levels in the tissues (see section 4.9.2.3).

7.6 Why mega quantities of vitamin C are beneficial to many individuals

It is apposite to summarize now the major arguments in favour of the need for consuming much higher quantities of ascorbate than those prescribed on the basis of the criteria of scurvy.

First, sub-clinical deficiency of vitamin C can be present in numerous individuals, despite ingestion of the recommended daily allowances of vitamin C.

·Secondly, higher intake is required prophylactically and more so therapeutically became many "normal" lives are nowadays under conditions of almost continuous biochemical stress which makes it necessary to

(a) meet ascorbate deficiencies arising from increased demands for the biosynthesis of neurohormones and in the attack of adreno-chrome, and

(b) ensure high blood-ascorbate levels and other tissue-ascorbate levels so as to ensure

   (i) higher efficiencies in ATP production and breakdown which are required for energy availability;

   (ii) upkeep of c-AMP levels by inhibition of over-activation of PDE;

   (iii) increased attack on bacteria by the white blood cells;

   (iv) increased γ-globulin biosynthesis (to offset antigen attack);

   (v) inhibition of over-activity of histamine, and

   (vi) enhanced formation of AFR as required.

---

* As early as 1936 Lojkin reported the deactivation of TMV in ascorbate solutions, provided they are aerated; this indicates formation of ascorbic free radicals.

Thirdly, higher intake is required than that computable in the first instance, because considerable oxidative degradation and deactivation by hydrolytic delactonization reduce the amount of ascorbate absorbed to very low proportions.

However, not all individuals require mega intake. This depends on the extent of physiological response to biochemical stress, to the extent to which the diet assists the deactivation of ascorbate, and to the extent that the individual can biosynthesize ascorbate (see Chapter 8).

7.7. The medical potential of vitamin C

There are numerous malfunctions and malaises which can be judged to derive benefit from mega vitamin C administration. The experimental/medical evidence obtained has often been conflicting. This more often than not was due to insufficiently large dosage and inadequate control of diet and timing. To consider all these would require a tome. A number of malfunctions and malaises have been considered in Chapter 4. Others such as nervous strain, the common cold, some viral attacks, cancer and some cardiovascular malfunctions are considered here. The principles outlined previously can be equally well applied to other malfunctions and malaises.

7.7.1. Nervous strain (see also section 4.10.2)

Worry, excitement, fear, anger and the "rat-race" are psychological factors which necessitate increased neurotransmitter activity, thus involving increased biosynthesis and utilization (followed by destruction) of the neurotransmitters noradrenaline, adrenaline, and serotonin. All these require ascorbate at one stage or another for their biosynthesis and protection from oxidation (see Chapter 4), and, to allow for inevitable losses, correspondingly more ascorbate is required for replenishment.

The activities of several other hormones are mediated via c-AMP. The formation of c-AMP follows potentiation of adenylcyclase which is activated by catecholamines such as adrenaline (see Chapters 2 and 4). If ascorbate levels are depleted as a result of increased biosynthesis of noradrenaline and serotonin, c-AMP will subsequently be biosynthesized to a smaller extent resulting in lower c-AMP levels; indeed, lower c-AMP levels are associated with depressed mental states (see section 4.10.2). Further, for a given PDE concentration, the lower the ascorbate levels, the more PDE sites should be free for hydrolytic attack on c-AMP. Thus lowered ascorbate levels result in neglect of two pathways which contribute to the maintenance of c-AMP levels.

Increased formation of noradrenaline and adrenaline increases the probability of leakage into other tissues and subsequent oxidation of adrenochrome and noradrenochrome which are highly toxic (see sections 2.2.5 and 4.3.2). Ascorbate encountering these chromes will reduce/deactivate them. Some would be lost in the process, thus causing ascorbate depletion unless the supply of ascorbate is abundant. This approach is accommodated by the finding that traumatic shock causes a transitory fall in plasma ascorbate. The transitory nature of the fall can be explained by rapid utilization and subsequent release of ascorbate from its storage sites, such as in the adrenals.

The beneficial effects following administration of very high daily doses of ascorbic acid to schizophrenic patients (e.g. Hoffer and Osmond, 1963, 1967)—in whom sudden brain activities can produce abnormally high adrenaline and adrenochrome concentrations—can be accommodated within the framework of detoxification of adrenochrome by ascorbate. It is apposite to note the findings (Briggs, 1962; Vander Kamp, 1966; Hoffer and Osmond, 1967) that schizophrenics can metabolize much more of vitamin C than normal individuals, and that serum ascorbate levels in schizophrenics were significantly lower than those of normal individuals (e.g. Ackerfeldt, 1957).

7.7.2. The common cold, influenza, sinusitis and associated malaises of the respiratory system

7.7.2.1. *Overview*

There have been various reports in the literature describing investigations on the effect of higher daily intake of ascorbate/ascorbic acid in respect of prophylaxis and therapy of the "common cold". Some of the conclusions are negative, some are non-committal, and some are positive in that they consider that there has been some or considerable improvement in the severity and/or reduction of the duration of the upsets of the individual subject to the common cold. Incidence, type, duration and severity of the attacks have been used as criteria in most of the investigations. A list of the published researches with some relevant breakdown is given in

Table 7.1. Conflicting conclusions have been arrived at in various reviews. It is not proposed to examine each of the investigations in detail.

An overall evaluation will be presented later on, but in the meantime it must be stressed that none of these investigations has:

(a) attempted to relate the results to c-AMP levels or to inhibition of PDE during the experimental period;

(b) evaluated the relative concentrations of ascorbate and of Del-A in blood or in the leucocytes, or in the respiratory system;

(c) eliminated any placebo effects by dividing the patients into the three groups of (i) non-placebo control, (ii) placebo-administered, and (iii) vitamin C administered and

(d) taken into account the time/diet factors which can have a controlling role in the protection or destruction of the vitamin.

(a) and (b) obviously could not have been attempted because of the then unappreciated relationship between ascorbate PDE inhibition and c-AMP and of the significance of Del-A. (c) unfortunately, was also not appreciated. However, many so-called placebos which are presumed to be without effect definitely do have some.* Thus, lactate complexes with Mg^{++} and by removing the ionic Mg^{++}—essential for PDE activity—can effectively depress or eliminate the activity of this enzyme in the decomposed bacterial flora in the intestine, thereby enhancing escape of ascorbate present in the food from deactivation to Del-A.†

I have proposed (Lewin, 1974c and e) that higher ascorbate concentrations should result in increased c-AMP levels. This was confirmed by van Wyk and Kotze (1975) and Tisdale (1975). Re-investigation of the effects of ascorbate levels in terms of c-AMP levels and associated effects of the common cold, is called for.

I shall describe—albeit briefly—my own discomfort in respect of the common cold and of allied ailments until I started taking mega quantities of vitamin C. From childhood to 1968 I suffered repeatedly from frequent attacks of nasal stuffiness, sinusitis, colds, sore throats, catarrh and associated respiratory malaises and discomforts.

---

* It is relevant that the use of placebo tablets in the case of tests on bacterial viruses in infection in asthma have led to improvement in 52.5% of the cases (Fontana et al., 1965); see also Frankland et al. (1955).

† Some groups of participants were given placebos containing lactose or citric acid. A number of intestinal bacteria ferment lactose to lactic acid which—by complexing with Mg^{++}—enhances the escape of ascorbate from deactivation by PDE thereby blurring the levels of ascorbate absorbed by the different groups; citrates also complex with Mg^{++}.

Table 7.1. Effect of vitamin C on the common cold and allied respiratory malaises

Investigators	Year	Type of participants	Daily dose (G)	Type of control (blind)	Ascorbate or ascorbic	Tablets or powder	Ascorbate content of blood	Attackers determination bacteria viruses	Interpretation
Cowan et al.	1942	Students	0.2 to 0.5	Single blind	Acid	Tablets	—	C.C.	Slight benefits, mainly no benefit
Glazebrook and Thomson	1942	Adolescents	Up to 0.2	—	Acid	Powder or tablets	—	C.C.	Practically no benefit
Markwell	1947	General population	0.75	—	Acid	N.S.	—	C.C.	Beneficial
Caels	1953	General population	10	—	Acid	Syrupy solution	—	C.C.	Some benefit (general well-being)
Franz et al.	1956	Medical students and nurses	3 × 0.065	Single blind	Acid	Capsules	Determined	C.C.	Beneficial
Ritzel	1961	Adults (skiers)	1.0	Single blind	Acid	Tablets	—	C.C.	Beneficial
Barnes	1961	High school pupils	0.2	—	N.S.	Multivitamin tablets	—	C.C.	Multivitamin tablets with vit. C: beneficial
Banks	1965	Personnel of firms	N.S.	Double blind	N.S.	Capsules	—	C.C.	Beneficial
Walker et al.	1967	Adults	3.0	Single blind	Effervescent	Tablets	—	Several viruses innoculated	
Regnier	1968	General population	0.6 every 3 hrs	Double single blind	Ascorbic acid	Powder	—	C.C.	Beneficial

General practitioner	1968	Medical practitioners and families	3 x 1	Double blind	Effervescent	Tablets	—	C.C.	No benefit
Anderson et al.	1972	General population	1.0	Double blind	Ascorbate	Tablets	—	C.C.	Some benefit
Charleston and Clegg	1972	Students and lecturers	1.0	Single blind	—	Tablets	—	—	Beneficial
Cheraskin et al.	1973	Medical practitioners and wives	0.2 to 0.4	N.S.	N.S.	N.S.	—	C.C.	Beneficial
Schwartz et al.	1973	Adult male prisoners	3 x 1	Double blind	Acid	Tablets	Determined	Rhino virus 44	No benefit
Wilson and Loh	1973	Boys and girls' schools and students	0.2 to 0.5	Single blind	Acid	Tablets	Determined	C.C.	Beneficial
Coulehan et al.	1974	School children	1 and 2 g	Double blind	Acid	Tablets	Determined	C.C.	Beneficial
Anderson et al.	1974	General population	0.25 to 8	Double blind	Ascorbate	Tablets	—	C.C.	Beneficial at highest doses
Karlowski et al.	1974	Adults	3 to 6	Mainly double blind	Ascorbate	Capsules	—	C.C.	Some benefit

N.S. = Not stated
C.C. = Common cold

The colds caught were often very heavy, and the discomforts associated with a blocked, stuffy nose often made breathing by mouth inescapable. Relief was obtained by using medicaments containing menthol and eucalyptus and aspirin; and ephedrine drops were often used, sometimes replaced by benzedrine inhalers when these became available.

Since following the mega vitamin C ingestion (*c*. 2 to 3 g total of three daily doses) which was started unintentionally as a result of my wife buying 1 g effervescent ascorbate tablets in 1968, I have had fewer colds each year, and their severity and duration has been significantly smaller. I can still induce an attack of a cold by exposure to suitable conditions or by contact with individuals with colds. However, the symptoms of the colds are less severe than those I was accustomed to prior to the mega ascorbic regime. Further, I can greatly depress the severity and duration of the symptoms by increasing the dosage to *c*. $\frac{3}{4}$ to 1 g of ascorbic acid every hour or so during the day, and the following day if necessary, within a couple of hours of the attack starting. The last provision is most important, since the later one applies the regime of *c*. 1 g every hour or so the less effective does the treatment become. It is also important not to expose oneself to further adverse conditions during the treatment, if maximum benefit is to be obtained.

Consider the mass of conflicting evidence and associated para- doxes in the results of investigation of the intake of mega quantities of vitamin C in respect of prophylaxis and therapy of the common cold. It seems to me that the population as a whole can be subdivided into a number of groups in respect of their ability to utilize ascorbate prophylaxis and therapy, and that the physiological differences can be such as to blur the significance of the clinical results.

At one end of the scale there are those who are prone to bacterial and viral attacks and who are exposed to respiratory ailments because they do not possess the capacity to resist the attacking agents. In such individuals mega vitamin C prophylaxis, although not absolute, is nevertheless definitely operative provided care is taken to reduce degradation and deactivation of the administered ascorbate prior to its absorption; at the onset of a cold the therapy conferred by immediate increase of the intake to *c*. 1 g every hour is invaluable. These individuals normally appear incapable of raising their antibody and interferon production to overcome the attacks in absence of mega vitamin C administration. Also they mostly do not suffer gastrointestinal discomforts on ingesting mega quantities of vitamin

C. Mega vitamin C intake ensures a clear increase in the ability to withstand bacterial/viral attacks and also to act in an anti-histamine capacity, thus giving relief in conditions associated with endogenous over-production and release of histamine into the vascular system. The mechanism by which the increased levels of ascorbate can be visualized to be expressed comprise inhibition/retardation of the depression of c-AMP levels by PDE, resulting also in small increases in the c-AMP levels and associated medical benefits. This consideration applies also to individuals who are adversely affected by gastrointestinal effects following mega administration of vitamin C (e.g. diarrhoea and excessive gas formation; Regnier, 1968). Such discomforts can often be overcome by anti gas formation treatment, such as the use of methyl-cellulose (c. 2.5 g three times daily).

In my own experience 64 (out of 69) individuals who had suffered considerable discomfort associated with the respiratory system noticed significant relief on undertaking mega ingestion of vitamin C.* When advised that the long-term effects of mega intake of vitamin C are not established in all individuals,† and that if they wished to abandon the mega intake of vitamin C at a later date they should do so gradually, the almost invariable response was that in view of the improvement they had undergone they simply could not face returning to their previous sufferings.

At the other end of the scale there are those individuals who are not—or do not appear to be—in need of mega vitamin C intake. This non-requirement may be due to intrinsic ability to biosynthesize ascorbate to a much greater extent than other individuals and/or the possession of physiological regulatory systems in which c-AMP levels are readily maintained or raised without much dependence on ascorbate levels. This may be due in part to a lower PDE activity or a more efficient control of it.

The question naturally arises as to why a regimen of an ingestion of c. 1 g of vitamin C is required about every hour, and why it is necessary to start this regimen at the first indication that a cold is coming on. To understand this it is necessary to appreciate the involvement of three factors in the development of the cold and relevant treatment by vitamin C, namely the initial cause, the

---

* These individuals did not experience any adverse gastrointestinal discomforts on taking mega quantities of vitamin C. Five individuals who experienced such discomforts did not proceed with the investigation.

† In view of the considerable experiences of Klenner (1971), Hoffer (1973) and of Poser (1972) it appears unlikely that there are any deleterious effects.

sequence of bacterial/viral multiplication and the maintenance of high ascorbate levels in the blood.

7.7.2.2. *The initial cause of the cold, and the sequence of bacterial/ viral multiplication*

The common cold can usually be initiated in two different ways; the associated effects are schematically illustrated in Fig. 7.1. One is to expose the individual to low-temperature conditions, such as cold winds, as a result of which the respiratory system is chilled, thereby resulting in disordered hormone balance followed in a vicious circle by decreased c-AMP levels and decreased antibody and interferon production. The resultant overcoming by the originally quiescent bacterial/viral agents, present in the respiratory tract, of the existing antibodies and interferon gives rein to the development of the cold. It is reasonable to assume that the early stages in bacterial/viral multiplications are more subject than others to adverse effect by high ascorbate levels. Provided sufficiently high levels of ascorbate are present in the blood and in the respiratory tract *in time* for ensuring increased resistance to the bacterial/viral attack, the attack is likely to be overcome.

A second way is to expose the individual to an atmosphere where infection by highly active bacteria and viruses in sneeze droplets is likely. Here the disorganization of the normal pattern of enzyme activity is followed by disturbance of the hormone balance and the resultant vicious circle, as a result of which the bacterial/viral attack gains momentum. Here again bacterial/viral multiplication has probably its Achilles' heel in its sequence; the early development may be more susceptible to high ascorbate levels. When catarrhal conditions are allowed to develop they probably inhibit the high levels of aeration required for the formation of ascorbic free radicals.*

It is apposite to consider the negative results of ascorbate treatment in the three investigations in which infection was caused by nasal instillation of virus cultures (Walker *et al.*, 1967; Hornick, 1972; Schwartz *et al.*, 1973). This method of infection is so markedly different from the normal sneeze-infection that it is surprising that the difference has not been stressed before. The nose-droplets in the sneezing of humans are likely to contain some antibodies which are enmeshed in mucus. The mucus would tend to

---

* Murata (1975) and Murata and Kitagawa (1973) have observed that ascorbate in aerated conditions *in vitro* has a virucidal action which has been demonstrated by studies on a number of phages.

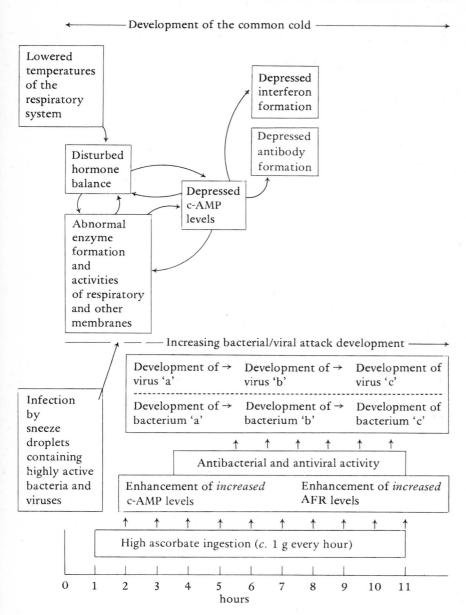

Fig. 7.1. Schematic representation of the malfunctioning of physiological activities with development of the common cold, and therapeutic impact of mega ascorbic administration.

arrest viral movement; thus the sneeze-droplets are unlikely to be ideal media for promotion of attack. Nasal instillation from laboratory cultures contain ideal media for viral development, thereby enhancing attack. Thus two factors blotted out the potential of ascorbate in fighting infection. First, a contrived and more powerful method of infection was used. Second, the full potential of ascorbate available in 1 g hourly ingestion was not realized; only a daily total intake of 3 g was employed, and as a result maximum ascorbate levels in the plasma and respiratory tract were not attained.

I would suggest that the use of ascorbate solutions for spraying into the respiratory system be investigated with a view to utilization in combating the common cold and associated malaises.

7.7.2.3. *The maintenance of high ascorbate levels in the blood and in the respiratory system*

High ascorbate levels in the blood—and particularly in the respiratory tissues—can be reached and maintained provided ascorbic acid in quantities of about 1 g is ingested at approximately one and a half hour intervals; the highest recorded ascorbate values in blood are between 2.2 mg and 3 mg per 100 ml of the serum (e.g. Lowry *et al.*, 1952; Linkswiler, 1958; Rhead and Schrauzer, 1971; Coulehan, 1974).* When 1 g is taken every hour for nine hours they can attain almost 4 mg %.† This is so because the initial upsurge in ascorbate concentration is temporary as a result of the renal threshhold in ascorbate excretion when steady state levels are reached following a balance between rate of absorption into the blood stream and rate of removal by the glomeruli.‡ If no frequent additions are made to compensate for the loss of the ascorbate (and permit uptake by other tissues) the maximum reached after about two to three hours is reduced to lower levels *c.* 0.4 to 0.9 mg per 100 ml of serum) after two or more hours.§ The effect of frequent "topping up" of the ascorbate can be represented as in Fig. 7.2. The asymptotic nature of the maximal levels of ascorbate in the blood following mega

---

* Still higher ascorbate concentrations in blood serum can be attained by intravenous infusion of ascorbate. Thus Masek and Hruba (1964) obtained in one patient, after intravenous infusion of 10 g ascorbate in 3 hours, ascorbate levels of 14 mg % and 91 mg % in serum and in leucocytes respectively.

† Lewin, S. Unpublished determinations.

‡ See section 6.2.4.

§ Several investigators have followed the variations in serum ascorbate levels after ascorbate ingestion (e.g. Todhunter *et al.*, 1942; Linkswiler, 1958). Although the time sequence deduced varies within 30 to 50% the overall pattern given above remains.

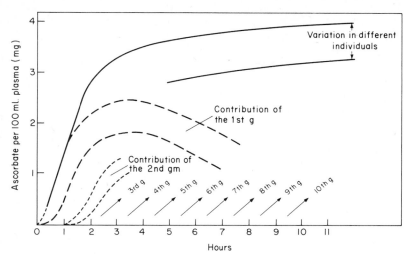

Fig. 7.2. Approximate variation of ascorbate levels in blood serum with hourly 1 g doses. (−) overall curve; others as indicated.

ingestion has been approximately computed taking into account various data in the literature (e.g. Todhunter *et al.*, 1942; Lowry *et al.*, 1952; Linkswiler, 1958; Masek and Hruba, 1964; Kübler and Gehler, 1970; Coulehan, 1974; and my unpublished data). The efficiency of the uptake is increased with increased frequency of ingestion of the ascorbic acid as the increased ascorbate levels favour increased uptake by the tissues, but is decreased by increased losses via the urine. The decreased efficiency of vitamin C absorption by the tissues with increased ingestion can be appreciated from Fig. 7.3.

The need for urgency in starting frequent mega ascorbate administration when a severe cold threatens is due to the interval before maximum ascorbate concentrations in the respiratory system are reached and the time that leucocytes and other defence agencies require to attain full activity; the interval is probably of the order of three to four hours. During this time the bacterial/viral activities become highly pronounced; therefore there is no time to be lost. Delay may well enable the attackers to become so powerful that rebuffing them becomes much more difficult.

It is relevant to consider another point in favour of the need for attainment of maximum ascorbate concentrations in blood and therefore in other human tissues. (Most other human tissues, including the respiratory system, contain higher ascorbate concentrations

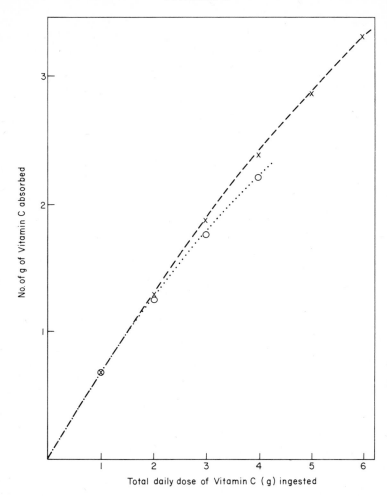

Fig. 7.3. Variation of the quantity of vitamin C absorbed with the amount ingested. (Plotted from data by Kubler and Gehler (1970) and recalculations by Mayersohn (1972).) X - - X total of 6 g in six equally distributed doses; O · · · · · O total of 4 g in four equally distributed doses.

than blood because of active transport.* *In vitro* it has been established that the minimum concentrations of ascorbate required to exhibit 25% inhibition of c-AMP phosphodiesterase (PDE) from

---

* The average concentration of ascorbate in the lungs of deceased humans over the age range of 1 year to 77 years was found to be between 5.8 and 4.5 mg per 100 g of lung tissue (Yavorsky *et al.*, 1934). This indicates a significantly higher concentration that that present in human serum.

beef heart is 10^{-4} M (Moffat *et al.*, 1972); and it would be expected that higher concentrations would result in even greater inhibition; this has proved to be the case (see Chapter 3). Frequent ingestion of *c*. 1 g ascorbate does ensure higher ascorbate levels in blood, and correspondingly should ensure still higher levels in the respiratory system, thereby inhibiting PDE more strongly and thus assisting in the maintenance of the required c-AMP level.

It is interesting to compare the effect of other substances which are used in treating the common cold in respect of their inhibition potential on PDE activity. Aspirin (acetylsalicylic acid), caffeine, paracetamol and codeine phosphate are frequently used individually or in combination for treating the common cold. These four compounds exhibit 25% PDE inhibition at 10^{-3} M concentration in comparison with ascorbate which requires only 10^{-4} M for the same percentage inhibition (Moffat *et al.*, 1972). Thus ascorbate is a more efficient PDE inhibitor, and no doubt a safer one.

7.7.3. Herpes

Herpes comprise a group of viruses the attacks of which give rise to various symptoms in humans. Three classes of associated malaises are usually recognized.

*Cold sores.** These are blister-like inflammations on the lips which although causing discomfort and highly irritating, are not serious, and usually last from four to eight days. They often follow catarrhal conditions as well as other skin irritations.

Shingles—often termed herpes zoster—which are associated with inflammation of parts of the nervous system.

Genital herpes† which are symptomatically somewhat similar to cold sores but which are localized on the genitals; they are considered to be carcinogenic (see also section 9.4.3).

Inactivation of herpes virus by mega intake of vitamin C has been reported by Holden and Resnick (1936), Holden and Molloy (1937), Dainow (1943), Klenner (1949) and Zureick (1950). Such inactivation can be understood on the lines that sufficiently high levels of ascorbic free radicals can be produced by highly aerateable conditions involving high ascorbate concentrations which can then cause single-strand DNA scission—as indicated by the results of Murata *et*

---

* Often referred to in the literature as herpes virus type 1.
† Often referred to in the literature as herpes virus type 2.

al. (1973, 1975) and possibly also by local ascorbate inactivation of catalase thereby raising the local H_2O_2 levels to ranges which are likely to be lethal to the viruses present.

I have confirmed the beneficial effects of mega vitamin C administration (using oral ingestion) in 38 individuals who were regularly subject to heavy attacks of "cold sores" three to five times yearly for several years and thus represented ideal "hard" cases. Following a total intake of 1 to 2 g ascorbic acid daily, the following were noted over a period of four years of vitamin C intake in each individual.

Thirty individuals had *no* subsequent attacks of herpes, the remaining eight had one or two attacks in which the duration and severity (number and size of blisters) were greatly reduced. Six of these eight individuals subsequently tried increased ascorbic acid daily administration of four to five times daily doses each of *c.* $\frac{3}{4}$ g of ascorbic acid as soon as the first tenderness on the lips was noted. In all these eight cases, the result was inhibition of blister development and disappearance of the tenderness within a day or two. Admittedly there were no double-blind trials, but in such "hard" cases the benefits obtained were so pronounced that the individuals needed no further convincing.

7.7.4. Other virus-caused malaises

There are various conflicting reports in the literature concerning the use of mega vitamin C administration in a number of virus-caused illnesses such as poliomyelitis, virus pneumonia and hepatitis. The results of Dalton (1962), Klenner (1959) and Jugenblut (1935, 1937, 1939) were mainly favourable. Knight and Stanley (1944) reported virucidal effects of 5×10^{-2} M ascorbic acid on influenza virus, and Baur and Staub (1954) observed beneficial effects in the case of hepatitis; their conclusions were confirmed by Kirchmair and Kirsch (1957). On the other hand Sabin (1939) eventually concluded that the beneficial effects could not be reproduced. Versteeg (1969)—using a system of mouse embryo cell cultures *in vitro*—concluded that ascorbate has no effect on Semliki Forest virus replication, and production and activity of interferon. However his highest ascorbate concentrations were 6 mg per 100 ml of medium, i.e. a concentration of 3×10^{-4} M (which were very much lower than those of Knight and Stanley (1944)); also his media were not effectively aerated.

7.7.5. Malfunctions of the cardiovascular system

7.7.5.1. *Overview*

Cardiovascular defects comprise a number of malfunctions. They can be physical in origin, e.g. weakened muscles or valves or heavily calcified fatty deposits in the intima of the arteries; or physiological in origin, e.g. overlengthy vasoconstriction (of the blood vessels leading to the heart muscle) which can be caused by excessive secretion of histamine and which can result in symptoms of angina pectoris. Atherosclerosis is associated with thickening of the arteries and with high levels of cholesterol in the blood (and its deposition in the intima).

Damage to the collagen matrix of the muscles may readily be rectified when plentiful supply of ascorbate is available. Heart muscle stores less ascorbate than other tissues except plasma—see Table 4.1—but the need for plentiful supply of ascorbate appears to be met by the leucocytes in the abundant blood vessel distribution which pervades the heart muscles. It is relevant to draw attention to the observations of Hume *et al.* (1972) that the ascorbate levels of leucocytes in 31 patients who had sustained an acute myocardial infarction were reduced to scorbutic levels within 12 hours of the infarctions. These events were related to the size of the myocardial infarction as reflected by serum aspartate aminotransferase levels. It is worthwhile correlating these observations with those of Srivastava and Sirohi (1969) that ascorbate reduces the activity of the three transaminating enzymes of glutamate-glyoxalate, glutamate-oxaloacetate and alanine-glyoxalate. If ascorbate is effective in decrease of these aminotransferase activities because it helps to repair the damage caused by membrane breakdown in the ruptured cells (and thus reduces seepage of the aminotransferases) then the need for replenishment of ascorbate levels, as they are rapidly used, explains the usefulness of mega ascorbate administration in myocardial infarctions.

It must be stressed that—as in other malfunctions/malaises—mega vitamin C intake, although useful, is by no means a panacea for cardiovascular defects. Cardiovascular malfunctions can arise from defective coordination of nervous impulses for which hardly any beneficial contribution may be expected from plentiful supply of ascorbate. Similarly hypertension (and associated high blood pressure) can originate in malfunctions which cannot be wholly ameliorated by high ascorbate intake or by higher c-AMP levels. Thus, in some individuals treatment by diuretics only is sufficient to over-come hypertension. Mega ascorbic acid ingestion does result in some diuresis (apparently because of the resultant higher acidity of the urine).* However, the degree of diuresis obtained does not match the higher levels of diuresis attainable by the use of special diuretics.

7.7.5.2. Angina

Angina pectoris is characterized by shortness of breath accom-panied by a "chest pain" caused by an insufficient supply of oxygen to meet the requirements of the heart-muscle. The insufficiency can originate in restriction of the blood flow to the heart-muscle by decreased diameter of the arteries/arterioles thereby decreasing the quantity of blood per second entering the muscle area. This can result from the development of "furry deposits" in the arteries, and from over-contraction of the smooth muscle of the walls of the arteries/arterioles (which effect can be caused by histamine). Relax-ation of the smooth muscle, on the other hand, results in increased blood flow.

Inhibition of increased PDE activity by inhibitory agents (such as methylxanthine and papaverine) has been reported to enhance relaxation of smooth muscle activity. Two factors are involved: c-AMP is known to play a role in (i) the IgE-mediated release of histamine† and (ii) in the adrenergic-mediated relaxation of smooth muscle.‡ These two activities have been considered to act in concert to reduce the release of histamine while favouring the adrenergic substances in a smooth muscle relaxing activity. Also, contractions of intestinal smooth muscle are inhibited by large concentrations of vitamin C (Dawson et al., 1967; Dawson and West, 1965).

Inhibition of constriction of blood supply to heart muscle would also be attained by reducing adrenaline or noradrenaline activity, as a result of association with ascorbate, since such complex formation should reduce the ability of these hormones to induce constriction of cardiac smooth muscle. Increased Ca^{++} availability is probably also involved in anginal trends. Ca^{++} entry into the muscle is a requisite for muscular contraction; relaxation of the muscle occurs on exit of

---

* e.g. Shaffer et al. (1944); Kenway et al. (1952).

† For several references see Austen and Lichtenstein (1973).

‡ β-adrenergic substances have been shown to induce the relaxation of smooth muscle preparations and also to favour a rise in c-AMP levels in these muscles (e.g. Polacek and Daniel, 1971; Angles d'Auriac and Meyer, 1972; Anderson and Nilsson, 1972). For numerous references see also Schultz et al. (1973).

the Ca^{++}. Hence raised Ca^{++} concentration levels should—by favouring prolongation of contraction—assist in restriction of blood supply and thereby enhance angina (see also section 9.4.4).

I have followed mega administration in ten individuals subject to anginal phenomena. I have noted that an intake of several 1 g daily doses of ascorbic acid/ascorbate is accompanied by decreased proneness to angina in these individuals. The beneficial effects appeared to comprise both transient and long-term influences.

Transient effects. Within an hour or so of ingestion of 1 g of the vitamin the individuals could undertake those light efforts such as bending and lifting small weights much more easily without bringing on anginal symptoms. This improvement lasted for two to three hours only. Another dose of *c.* 0.7 or 1 g would bring on further relief for a similar period.

Long term. Taken over a year and longer, the proneness to anginal incidence decreased gradually. There was much less need for glycerol-trinitrate tablets which had been required when taking a walk of a mile or two. Eventually, in many cases they could be dispensed with.

The prophylactic effect of ascorbate can be understood in terms of the ability of high ascorbate levels in the tissues to inhibit (i) increased PDE activity, (ii) effects of histamine over-activity, and (iii) the constrictive effect of adrenaline/noradrenaline on smooth muscle. The long-term therapeutic effect can be explained in terms of increased probability of dissolution of the arterial deposits; see also section 4.8.1.

7.7.5.3. Atherosclerosis and implication of cholesterol levels in relation to ascorbate concentration levels

Current paradoxes in influence of mega ascorbate intake on atherosclerosis and associated cholesterol levels. Atherosclerosis is often characterized by lesions of fatty thickening (containing cholesterol and lipds) of the intima of certain arteries. The existence of a relationship between ascorbate deficiency in the arteries and lipid deposition in the arteries of apparently well-nourished individuals has been indicated by the results of Becker *et al.* (1953), Willis (1957) and Willis and Fishman (1958) and has led to the preliminary conclusion that a high concentration of ascorbate is essential for the prevention of atherosclerosis, although at the time no determinations were made as to the influence of ascorbate on blood cholesterol levels (see also Sokoloff *et al.* (1966) for a review).

High cholesterol levels in the blood have often been implicated in the development of hypertension and coronary disease. The literature over the past thirty years contains several publications with conflicting conclusions as to the effect of higher ascorbate intakes on cholesterol levels in the blood. A representative sample is given in Table 7.2 for illustration, along with some breakdown.

The conflicting conclusions may have resulted from the following:

Diet. The effect of diet on deactivation and delactonization of the ingested ascorbate can be a controlling factor. This has been considered in detail previously.

Late stage of the malaise. The longer the period during which atherosclerosis has progressed the longer the period and the greater the dosage of ascorbate administration required. Also the damage caused to the repair mechanisms may have attained such levels that controls which would have benefited from mega ascorbate intake are no longer effective.

Mg^{++}/Ca^{++} in absorption. Many cases have been traced where atherosclerosis appears to have been favoured by high Ca^{++}/Mg^{++} ratios in drinking water. In such cases mega ascorbate administration is likely to prove very useful.

There is considerable evidence that the probability of coronary malfunction is lower in hard-water than in soft-water districts (e.g. Bloch, 1973). Since coronary malfunction is enhanced by formation of calcified deposits in the cardiovascular system; and since hard-water contains significantly high proportions of calcium salts, this introduces a paradox. It has already been suggested that the prophylactic effect of hard-water is associated with increased proportion of magnesium to calcium in it. I wish to propose a simple explanation to the phenomenon, in terms of the experimentally established greater solubility of magnesium deposits as compared to the calcium analogues.

Arterial deposits consist mainly of Ca/phospholipid/cholesterol complexes. When magnesium is present in significant proportions, the following interchange should take place:

$$Ca/phospholipid/cholesterol + Mg^{++} \rightleftharpoons$$

$$Ca^{++} + Mg/phospholipid/cholesterol$$

Mg salts possess greater solubility than their corresponding Ca complexes. Hence the formation of the Mg complex should enhance decreased arterial deposits. Currently we are engaged in an investigation on the effect of a combination of Mg^{++} salts (in presence of

Table 7.2. Effect of mega ascorbic administration on blood fat and cholesterol levels

Investigator	Year	Ascorbate dose (g) daily	Oral or intravenous	Blood fat levels	Cholesterol level	Type of patient	Conclusion
Tiapiana	1952	0.5 daily for several weeks	Intravenous	–	Lowered	Coronary disease	Method effective
Lobova	1953	1.0 for 10 days	Intravenous	β-proteins lowered; α-proteins raised in 18 of 35 patients	–	Coronary disease	Responding patients were in early phase of the disease
Anderson et al.	1958	1 g	Oral		No significant lowering	Having between 160 and 200 mg% cholesterol levels	Negative results obtained probably do not contradict results obtained by others at over 200 mg% cholesterol
Samuel and Ohalchi	1964	2 x (0.5 to 3) 5 to 16 weeks	Oral, but 2 patients on 0.5 g intravenous injections for 2–4 weeks	–	No noticeable difference except in one patient	14 patients with over 300 mg% cholesterol	Mega ascorbate administration does not reduce cholesterol but some patients benefited
Sokoloff et al.	1966	1.5 2–3	Oral Oral	Not lowered Lowered	Not lowered	Pronounced hyper cholesteremia	Most patients benefited
Ginter et al.	1970	3 x 0.1	Oral	–	After 47 days levels decreased	Village population	Effect most pronounced in persons with hyper cholesteremia
Spittle	1971	1	Oral	–	Variable	Various	Any rise in serum cholesterol observed was considered due to mobilization of arterially deposited cholesterol
Myasnikov	1958	0.1 to 0.2 per rabbit		Lowered	Lowered	Rabbits	Atherosclerosis retarded

physiologically acceptable chelating agents) and ascorbate on a number of malaises (see section 9.4.4).

c-AMP and cholesterol levels. As pointed out by Butcher *et al.* (1970), c-AMP potentiates the metabolism of cholesterol to pregnenolone in the adrenal cortex, the corpus luteum, the ovaries and testis, thus

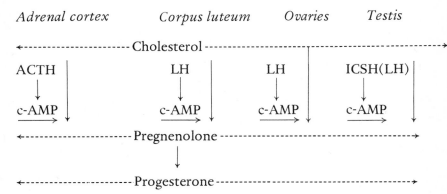

Adrenal cortex   *Corpus luteum*   *Ovaries*   *Testis*

Cholesterol levels are the result of a "steady state" effect in which control is exercised by input and metabolism, thus

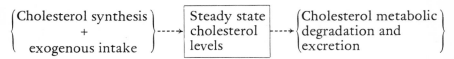

The activity of high intake of ascorbate in respect of contribution to the lowering of cholesterol levels can be understood in terms of its influence on c-AMP levels, as discussed previously. However, release of cholesterol from the walls of the vessels, and increased biosynthesis and ingestion of cholesterol are bound to blur any expected reduction in cholesterol levels.

A complicating factor lies with variation due to biochemical individuality. In many individuals cholesterol metabolism is controlled mainly by c-AMP levels; in these cases high ascorbate levels are likely to be very useful. In other individuals much of the control of cholesterol mobilization and metabolism lies in other mechanisms; in these cases higher intake of ascorbate is unlikely to be effective (in so far as the influence of c-AMP levels is concerned). In view of these considerations it is essential to monitor c-AMP levels during mega ascorbate administration investigations. Unfortunately, this has not been carried out in past investigations.

7.7.6. Cancer and leukemia

7.7.6.1. *Overview*

A number of papers have been published which deal with the influence of vitamin C administration on the progress of malignancy *in vivo* and on cancerous cells *in vitro*. The results are conflicting. For several papers illustrating the conflicting conclusions see foot-note.* It is not feasible to carry out a meaningful analysis as to the reasons for the various results, because

(i) often the investigators used rather low ascorbic acid adminis-tration, such as up to only 0.2 g daily. This inference is lent support by the work of Goth and Littman (1948) who reported the most frequent incidence of cancer in tissues whose ascorbate levels were below 4.5% mg;

(ii) the method of intake of the vitamin has not been detailed;

(iii) the c-AMP levels have not been determined, and

(iv) the AFR levels have not been determined.

Of necessity we are restricted to a comparatively brief *overall* analysis of possible causes, effects and symptoms.

In any disease it is necessary to differentiate between the cause and the symptoms. Cancer is not a single disease but rather a number of conditions showing closely allied symptoms of malfunctions of the biological organization which manifest themselves in undisciplined cellular multiplication which intereferes with and eventually destroys the overall biological system. Cancerous con-ditions are known to arise from several causes such as the subjection to carcinogenic substances, attack by particular viruses, and exposure to high frequency radiation such as X-rays. The paradox of con-flicting results of ascorbate administration in cancer can be under-stood on the lines that some malignant activities respond favourably to high ascorbate levels by virtue of its ability to inhibit PDE, as well as its other, direct, beneficial activities such as those due to AFR, but that the prior development of the malaise can result in strong resistance to therapy.† The evidence that mega ascorbate intake has a

---

* Benade *et al.* (1969); McCormick (1954, 1963); Deucher (1940); Waldo and Zipf (1955); Klenner (1971); Vogt (1940); Plum and Thomsen (1936); Eufinger and Gaehtgens (1936); Szenes (1942); Picha and Weghaupt (1956); Schirmacher and Schneider (1955); Schneider (1954, 1955, 1956); Tagi-Zade (1961); Heinilid and Schiedt (1936); Kyhos *et al.* (1945).

† The strong resistance may be the result of the high consumption of oxygen by malignant tissues, as a result of which the oxygen tension is lowered to such an extent that formation of AFR is decimated.

beneficial influence on malignancy will be best considered in separate sections illustrating the effect of ascorbate on malignancy and the effect of c-AMP and PDE inhibitors on malignancy.

7.7.6.2. Ascorbate inhibition of carcinogens

The presence of carcinogens in the body can originate endogenously or exogenously. Sufficiently high intake of vitamin C has been shown to inhibit carcinogenic activities of certain substances. It is apposite to note that exposure of ascorbate-producing species to a number of carcinogenic substances results in multifold increases in the biosynthesis of the vitamin (see section 5.3.2). The potential of high ascorbate intake to inhibit carcinogens is illustrated in the following:

Endogenous development arising from faulty metabolism. 3-hydroxyanthranilic (3-HOA) has been shown to be carcinogenic in mice bladders (Allen *et al.*, 1957). Schlegel *et al.* (1969) studied the aetiology and prevention of bladder carcinoma; they concluded that the spontaneous oxidation of 3-HOA can be completely prevented by daily oral intake of 1.5 g of ascorbic acid.

Exogenous sources of carcinogens. Nitrosamines formed in acid conditions in the stomach (following intake of nitrites) are carcinogenic, but can be neutralized by large quantities of the vitamin (see section 4.8.3). Also anthracene and 3,4-benzpyrene (which are carcinogenic) can be detoxicated by ascorbic acid (Warren, 1943).

7.7.6.3. Deactivation of viruses filially related to viruses implicated in carcinogenesis

Ascorbate has been reported to inhibit the development of herpes viruses such as herpes zoster and shingle viruses (e.g. Holden and Molloy, 1937; Zureick, 1950; Klenner, 1951; Dainow, 1943; see also section 7.7.3). A member of the herpes family, i.e. the Epstein-Barr virus is believed to be implicated in African Burkitt's lymphoma and nasopharyngeal carcinoma, both of which give rise to lethal tumours in man. There is an association between herpes virus 2 and squamous cell carcinoma of the cervix (Rawls, 1973).

The herpes virus samiri causes cancer in primates (e.g. Laufs and Steinke, 1975). Since there is some indication that members of the herpes family are also adversely affected *in vivo* by high ascorbate levels, the possibility that other members can also be similarly affected cannot be excluded without corresponding trials.

Numerous viruses and bacteriophages have been reported to be deactivated by ascorbate in highly aerated conditions (e.g. Lojkin, 1938; Murata and Kitawage, 1973; see also sections 7.7.3 and 7.7.4).

7.7.6.4. *Ascorbate inhibition of cancerous cells* in vitro

Benade *et al.* (1969) have shown that ascorbate is extremely lethal to Ehrlich ascites carcinoma cells *in vitro*. Catalase and low oxygen tension were found to protect the cells from the lethal influence of ascorbate. The effect of ascorbate is probably influenced by its (limited) ability to deactivate catalase (see section 2.3.3). The "protective" effect of low oxygen tension is probably associated with the decreased probability of formation of AFR, since it has been demonstrated that the formation of AFR requires a high degree of aeration (see also section 7.7.2.2).

7.7.6.5. *Reduction of damage due to irradiation*

It has been reported (Deucher, 1940) that daily ingestion of up to 4 g of ascorbic acid results in significant beneficial effects in cancer patients, and in increased tolerance to irradiation with X-rays. Szenes (1942) concluded otherwise. However, the potential of AFR to scavenge free radicals of other species such as those formed by X-ray irradiation is nowadays appreciated; it is due to its antioxidant properties. In general, antioxidants have been found to scavenge X-ray radiation-induced free radicals (which otherwise can cause cancer) e.g. Tappel (1965). Szene's negative conclusions could therefore have been due to the use of highly developed cancer which was beyond reversal.

7.7.6.6. Modus operandi *of anti-malignancy activities of ascorbate*

From the above we can infer that ascorbate can exert—in some specific conditions—an anti-malignancy potential. Elucidation of the possible *modus operandi* of ascorbate on cancerous tissues should assist in disentangling the confusing web of ascorbate contents of tissues. In this connection it is pertinent to ask the following questions: If ascorbate has an anti-malignancy potential what ascorbate concentrations in malignant tissues are to be expected?

On the basis of the argument that ascorbate is utilized extensively in the mobilization of the body defence mechanisms against cancer, we would expect depletion of the ascorbate content of normal tissue, whether directly involved in defence or not, as the ascorbate is withdrawn for mobilization for the defence. However, the ascorbate content of tumour tissue may or may not be higher than that of its *normal parent* tissue, depending on the extent of active transport and the rate of utilization of ascorbate by the tumour tissue.* Consider in this light the available experimental data.

The expectation that the ascorbate reserves of an organism with a regular intake of ascorbate, under malignant attack, should be depleted as a whole is borne out by the results of Watson (1943) who established that the reserves of vitamin C in the guinea pig are soon exhausted by a rapidly growing tumour. Also, Gähtgens (1938) and Spellberg and Keeton (1939) reported vitamin C deficiency in patients suffering from cancer. However, in the case of rats—which species is capable of biosynthesizing vitamin C—Woodward (1935), Sure (1939), and Stepp and Schröder (1936) observed decreased vitamin C content levels in the organs of cancerous rats. The latter could result from damaged tissues no longer being able to respond by carrying out increased vitamin C biosynthesis.

So far we have considered whether ascorbate itself has a direct retarding influence on the progress of malignancy. However, if we reorient our thinking and rephrase our questions in terms of the influence of ascorbate on c-AMP levels, the pattern of events becomes clearer; c-AMP has been considered to have an adverse effect on the development of cancerous tissue *in vitro* and *in vivo*.

Gericke and Chandra (1969) reported inhibition of growth of subcutaneously transplanted lymphosarcoma in mice following injection of c-AMP.

Friedman and Pastan (1969) observed that the introduction of 10 mM of c-AMP resulted in significant increase in the antiviral activity of interferon in chick fibroblasts. Such antiviral activity could be influential in significant inhibition of virus induced carcinomas.

Pastan (reported in a personal communication by Butcher *et al.*, 1971) noted that c-AMP could cause some transformed cells in tissue culture to revert to a cell phenotype morphologically similar to untransformed cells.

Ryan and Heidrick (1969) reported that *in vitro* the growth of four tumorigenic cell lines was inhibited from 70 to 89% by 0.3 mM c-AMP, whereas a non-malignant cell line was only slightly affected.

---

* The report by Goth and Littman (1948) that in general tumours have higher concentration of vitamin C than their normal parent tissue indicates a very high transport requirement for rapidly developing tissue.

Oler, Iannacone and Gordon (1973) reported that the addition of dibutyryl c-AMP and theophylline to cultures of L cells resulted in inhibition of growth. Keller (1972) reported that substances which raise the level of intracellular c-AMP (by inhibition of PDE) suppressed tumour growth of Walker carcinoma in the rat.

If we follow the concept that c-AMP levels result from sufficiently high intake of vitamin C then—as in other malaises—the pattern of beneficial effect of high intake of the vitamin on malignant disease can be understood. As before allowance has to be made in respect of influences adversely affecting vitamin absorption as well as the original state of the malaise.

Future investigations as to the potential of ascorbate in cancer therapy must therefore include the monitoring of c-AMP levels, and of AFR levels.

It has been proposed by Cameron and Pauling (1973) that the ability of ascorbate to exert a beneficial influence on malignant disease is due to its activity on the hyaluronidase complex. Mammalian cells are normally emmeshed in intercellular glycosaminglycans which restrain them from increasing separation; depolymerization of the glycosaminglycans in the immediate vicinity of the cells would therefore release the cells from their cohesion. The enzyme hyaluronidase activates the depolymerization, but its activity is offset by a physiological hyaluronidase-inhibitor (PHI) which requires ascorbate for its biosynthesis. When the ascorbate levels are too low insufficient inhibitor activity exists, and this enables undisciplined proliferation to take place. So far there appears to be no experimental evidence in humans which favours or rejects this approach unequivocally. However, in the case of guinea pigs, it has been reported (Shapiro and Bishop, 1975) that PHI was not affected by ascorbic acid intakes as much as 1 g per kilo weight per day.

7.7.7. Are there any "side effects"?

7.7.7.1. Is there a limit to mega ascorbate administration because of "side-effects"?

There is general agreement that daily intake of ascorbic acid of c. 0.5 g for lengthy periods does not normally produce toxic effects. However, the administration of multi-gram quantities ranging from 1 g to 10 g daily has naturally raised the question whether the use of such mega quantities could give rise to undesirable side-effects. No matter how physiologically useful a substance is, there is always a range limit above which some adverse side-effects will be apparent. The upper limit of such a range differs with the substance, and the individual and his diet, age and medical history. The side-effects have to be balanced against the usefulness of the substance and the urgency of the particular treatment. Vitamins and other essential substances conform to this pattern, and there is no *a priori* reason as to why ascorbate should be an exception. It is the tacit acceptance of this concept that has probably caused several scientists to stress the hazard potential of mega vitamin C administration. Because of the lack of certainty that any substance will not cause physiological side-effects, it is necessary to consider this aspect of mega vitamin C administration as clearly as possible; let us therefore consider the various hazards mentioned in the literature and assess their potential.

7.7.7.2. *Is the formation of calcium oxalate calculi a real hazard?*

It is known that some of the ingested ascorbate is metabolized to oxalate (e.g. Lamden and Christokowski, 1954, 1971; Briggs *et al.*, 1973), and that it is mainly excreted in the urine.* It has been established that ingestion of ascorbate below 4 g daily results in average insignificant increases of oxalic acid excretion in the urine (Lamden and Christokowski, 1954†). It has been inferred that the greater the quantity of oxalate excreted, the greater should be the probability of calcium calculi formation and consequently the use of mega vitamin C administration should result in detrimental effects. Further, only one case of a healthy individual developing a urinal stone after taking a short course of ascorbic acid treatment has been reported (Briggs, 1973).

However, Klenner (1971), Poser (1972) and Hoffer (1973) have concluded from their wide experience over many years of prescribing multigram daily doses of ascorbic acid—when they noted no patients who suffered calcium oxalate stone formation—that such hazards are very remote. Also Takiguchi *et al.* (1966) found no significant increase in urinary oxalate excretion on administration of up to 2 g daily of ascorbic acid for up to 6 months; Murphy and Zelman (1965) also concluded after 3 years of investigation that the hazard of oxalate calculi formation is not significant.

---

* General information concerning formation of human stones is given by Lonsdale (1968) and by Gershoff (1964).

† At 8 g daily ingestion of ascorbic acid, the average increase was 1-fold.

Thus, the basic argument that an increase in oxalate excretion in the urine, resulting from mega intake of vitamin C, is likely to be accompanied by the formation of calcium oxalate stones is not valid; rather the reverse because of the accompanying increased acidity and increased ascorbate concentration in the urine.

(a) *Increased acidity*: Multigram administration of ascorbic acid is often recommended (McDonald and Murphy, 1959; Murphy and Zelman, 1965) for increased acidity of the urine which effect enhances bacteriostacis. Such acidity is exponentially effective in reducing calcium oxalate precipitation. This precipitation requires that the solubility product of $[Ca^{++}]\,[C_2C_4]$ be exceeded. Oxalic acid is a dibasic acid, and its ionization takes place in two stages. However, for the sake of simplicity we can write

$$H_2C_2O_4 \rightleftharpoons 2H^+ + C_2O_4^{--} \text{ and therefore } \frac{[C_2O_4^{--}]\,[H^+]^2}{[H_2C_2O_4]} = K.$$

Hence, increase in $[H^+]$ (the pH usually drops by about 0.5 to 1 pH units) should have an adverse effect to the second power on the $[C_2O_4^{--}]$, and correspondingly decreases the probability of calcium oxalate precipitation. Indeed, acid urine is known to solubilize calcium salts thereby reducing the hazard of stone formation (Hockaday and Smith, 1963).

(b) *Diuresis.** Stone formation requires *static* conditions when the initial minute nuclei, capable of passing through the fairly porous membranes of the kidney tissue, grow to larger sizes.† Diuresis by increasing urine flow obviates urolithiasis. Increasingly larger intakes of ascorbic acid are known to result in corresponding increases in diuresis; some physicians recommend as much as 10 g daily as a diuretic (e.g. Klenner, 1971). Increasing diuresis should therefore inhibit correspondingly the probability of stone formation.

(c) *Increased ascorbate concentration*: This results in increased complexing of the Ca^{++} thereby decreasing the free Ca^{++}. This decreases the probability of the solubility product of calcium oxalate being exceeded.

Hence increased ascorbic acid intake, although resulting in some increase in oxalic acid excretion in the urine, is hardly likely to increase the probability of the formation of calcium oxalate calculi.

---

* Abbassy (1937) and Kenaway *et al.* (1952) noted the diuretic effect of vitamin C and suggested its clinical use.

† Thus, formation of human stones was found to be prevented by Frank de Vries (1966) by increased drinking of water (and resulting urination).

7.7.7.3. Does mega ascorbic intake increase the probability of formation of uric acid stones?

The warning that mega intake of vitamin C is likely to result in increased probability of formation of uric acid calculi has been voiced on several occasions. It is therefore necessary to examine the available data. Intravenous (or intramuscular) injection of 0.5 g of vitamin C on two successive days in several patients resulted in the average values of uric acid in 6-hour urine of the subjects rising from 111 to 260 mg dropping subsequently to 102 mg. The corresponding average values for uric acid in the blood were 3.9, 4.1, 4.3 and 3.8 mg% (Pena *et al.*, 1963) (see also Pena *et al.*, Nutritional Abstracts and Reviews, 1964). The pattern is therefore that of an increase of *c.* 10% in uric acid concentration (following mega vitamin C administration*) together with a small increase in blood uric acid concentration; these are accompanied by approximately 1.5 times increase in the excretion of uric acid. Such a pattern suggests that any increase in vitamin C administration greatly potentiates uric acid excretion to an extent significantly greater than that of its increased blood levels. It is difficult to understand therefore how such data can reasonably be used to indicate increased probability of formation of uric acid calculi.

7.7.7.4. Gastrointestinal effects and discomforts

It has been stated in the literature (e.g. Goldsmith, 1971) that intake of daily 1 g ascorbic acid may cause diarrhoea; and Hume *et al.* (1973) reported that a total of 3 g daily resulted in most of the 7 patients experiencing abdominal colic and some looseness of the bowels. Regnier (1968) states that some heartburn can be caused in some individuals (and that this can be relieved by a small amount of bicarbonate), and that after several days of high vitamin C dosage excess abdominal gas formation may take place. This gas excess can reasonably be attributed to the reducing conditions enforced by higher concentrations of ascorbate favouring the predominance of anaerobic intestinal flora. I would suggest that the potential of increased ascorbate presence to favour the predominance of anaerobic flora could be due in part to the ability of the vitamin to

---

* It is apposite to point out that ascorbate absorption efficiency is very much greater in intravenous injection than in oral ingestion; thus an injection of 0.5 g of ascorbate is probably equivalent to an oral ingestion several times that quantity.

deactivate the breakdown by catalase of H_2O_2 (see also section 2.3.3). Anaerobic bacteria are highly susceptible to H_2O_2, because they are unable to form catalase. In the intestines the aerobic bacteria can withstand attack by H_2O_2 by virtue of the catalase they produce. This advantage is however lost, or considerably reduced, in the presence of comparatively high ascorbate concentrations when catalase activity is inhibited. Many individuals do not seem troubled by gas formation in spite of administration of high quantities of ascorbate. However, I have noted that those who are often so affected find respite when the vitamin is administered with meals, and particularly when they take methyl-cellulose (c. 2.5–3.5 g three times daily); both gas formation and discomfort are reduced to acceptable or barely noticeable levels. Some individuals found that the associated discomfort dropped to negligible levels on keeping the individual dose below 0.6 g or by taking slow-release vitamin C tablets. It is necessary to emphasize that many individuals who undergo mega vitamin C administration do not appear to be subject to this discomfort.

7.7.7.5. *Destruction of vitamin B12 by vitamin C*

The first reports that ascorbate tends to destroy vitamin B12 appeared some 20 years ago (Hutchins *et al.*, 1956). Later reports stated that oxidized vitamin B12 (with trivalent cobalt) is more stable than reduced vitamin B12 (with monovalent cobalt). Recently, Herbert and Jacob (1974) concluded that ascorbic acid can destroy vitamin B12 in food *in vitro* when the two are present simultaneously or *in vivo* within an hour before or after a meal. Also a considerable fraction of the 3 μg to 6 μg of vitamin B12 which is usually secreted daily in the bile would be destroyed before it could be resorbed in the intestines. The authors also considered that further destruction of vitamin B12 would take place in the blood by high ascorbate levels, when low daily intakes of c. 45 mg (recommended daily allowances) were used, but not when higher doses such as 0.5 g daily were administered, when as much as a third of vitamin B12 in human bile would be destroyed. Herbert and Jacob (1974) and Zuck and Connie (1963) noted that the presence of some iron salts decreases the destruction of vitamin B12.* Herbert and Jacob

---

* It is interesting that the decomposition products of aneurine (in solution at pH 8.0) and of aneurine and nicotinamide (at pH 4.5) and other reducing agents such as cysteine and H_2S destroy vitamin B12 activity, and that ferric chloride affords protection (Mukherjee and Sen, 1958).

(1974) suggested that the destruction of B12 can be reduced by taking the ascorbate two or more hours after the meal.

It is apposite to point out that the *in-vitro* experiments performed by Herbert and Jacob (1974) were carried out *without* the addition of HCl and the digestive enzymes necessary to mimic the conditions in the stomach; consequently the pH of the media is likely to have been neutral. They relied on preliminary control experiments only in which HCl was added. However, ascorbate in presence of air is oxidized far more readily than in acid conditions, thereby introducing another variable. It is therefore desirable to repeat the experiments under conditions which are indeed equivalent to those in the stomach in order to reach more certain conclusions as to the level of destruction of vitamin B12.

7.7.7.6. *Pentosuria*

Pentosuria is a condition in which the urine contains large quantities of the pentose L-xylulose and arabinose.* When large quantities of fruit or fruit juices are consumed, alimentary pentosurea is often encountered when the pentose ingested is excreted. Idiopathic pentosuria is an abnormality usually attributed to the congenital absence of L-xylulose dehydrogenase which reduces L-xylulose; as a result L-xylulose is excreted via the urine. There are no associated clinical syndromes.

Mašek and Hrubá (1964) observed that human subjects react to mega vitamin C intake with pentosuria. As xylulose reduces copper more readily than glucose, the pentosuria following mega vitamin C intake can result in mistaken diagnosis where diabetic mellitus tests are carried out. In such cases it is necessary to utilize enzymatic (glucose oxidase) tests.

7.7.7.7. *Infertility*

There have been several reports in the literature stating or inferring that mega vitamin C intake favours infertility or abortion (e.g. Briggs, 1973a, b; Samborskaja and Freedman, 1966). Ryan and Coronel (1969) reported inhibition of reproduction and ovulation when c-AMP was injected into female mice. It could be argued that mega

---

* It is interesting that in such persons intake of D-glucuronic acid results in considerable excretion of L-xylulose in the urine; this indicates that the xylulose pathway in the ascorbic/xylulose fork (see also Fig. 5.2) is heavily favoured in comparison with the ascorbic pathway.

ascorbate levels could under certain conditions increase c-AMP levels above normal to potentiate such effect. However, so far there is no evidence clearly pointing in this direction. Further, both Hoffer (1973) and Poser (1972) who have prescribed as many as 10 g daily of ascorbic acid to many patients have failed to observe such effect (see also Wilson and Loh, 1973).

7.7.7.8. *Interaction of ascorbate and warfarin*

Ascorbic acid administration has been reported to shorten the prothrombin time in animals receiving warfarin anti-coagulants (Sigell and Flessa, 1970) and in the case of one individual (Rosenthal, 1971; Hume *et al.*, 1972). In view of these reports, and until further confirmation or otherwise is obtained, patients who are undergoing warfarin administration should desist from mega vitamin C intake unless they do so under strict medical supervision.

7.7.7.9. *Diet and vitamin C administration*

There have been several reports in the literature (e.g. Patterson, 1949; Pillsbury *et al.*, 1973; Chatterjee, 1975) that ingestion by animals of mega quantities of vitamin C in carbohydrate-rich (and protein-poor) diets result in adverse effects such as increased DHA levels and increased mortality. The latter was often traced back to associated increases in blood sugar levels and to diabetes. These adverse effects were clearly dependent on low levels of protein in the diet. When protein formed a respectable proportion of the diet, these mishaps did not occur.

The increase in DHA can be understood on the lines that free Cu^{++} and iron ions present catalyse the oxidation of AA to DHA very rapidly, and that the DHA formed is the culprit since it has been shown (e.g. Patterson, 1951) that direct DHA administration results in fatal mishaps. When sufficient protein is present in the diet, the digested products, namely peptides and amino acids, should chelate the multivalent ions effectively, thereby inhibiting oxidation to DHA and also deactivation by PDE (from the intestinal flora) to the biologically inactive Del-A.

The undesirable effects resulting from protein-poor diets can therefore be avoided by ensuring that the mega vitamin administration takes place in presence of actual, or potential, acceptable chelating agents, or high protein diets.

7.7.7.10. *Rebound on sudden withdrawal of ascorbate*

There are several reports of adverse effects following sudden withdrawal from lengthy mega ascorbic intake, as well as of subsequent increased minimal requirements of ascorbate in terms of protection from scurvy, in humans and in guinea pigs (Jakowlew, 1958; Gordonoff, 1960; Rhead and Schrauzer, 1971). There have also been reports contradicting these conclusions in many individuals (e.g. Hoffer, 1973; Anderson *et al.*, 1974; Coulehan *et al.*, 1974). Thus biochemical individuality would appear to display its variability in this connection.

It is worthwhile pondering on the possible significance of this phenomenon. When some individuals have been subject to what might be termed "de-luxe" treatment with vitamin C and then are suddenly reduced to penury of this vitamin by having their intake cut down to, say, 50 mg daily, the physiology of the individual still continues to utilize the vitamin at the higher levels to which it has recently been accommodated, as a result the reserve pool of ascorbate could be rapidly depleted to scurvy levels.* In enzymatic terms the phenomenon can be pursued further. It has already been pointed out that many individuals are likely to biosynthesize their own vitamin C, albeit in quantities insufficient to meet even the minimal requirement. On a general level of discussion, we can use Le Chatelier's Principle to conclude that the higher ascorbate levels in the tissues would tend to affect adversely the last stage(s) of endogenous formation of ascorbate. A sudden cut-off in ascorbate supplies would thus not only decrease ascorbate availability, but leave ascorbate utilization and subsequent ascorbate metabolism to pentoses at the originally high "luxury" levels (unless given sufficient time for readjustment by very slow weaning off the ascorbate luxury usage) and thus would deplete the body of ascorbate reserves very quickly. It is therefore essential in the case of sensitive individuals to "retrain" the body to smaller availability of ascorbate gradually if physiological shocks are to be reduced to the minimum.

7.7.7.11. *Are there any possible adverse long-term effects?*

It is often argued that mega vitamin C administration of 2 to 10 g daily may involve unknown long-term adverse effects. However,

---

* When the ascorbate levels are high, it is quite possible that PDE biosynthesis and activity are enhanced, thereby utilizing the generous availability of ascorbate over-freely (see also Hrubá and Mašek, 1962).

numerous individuals have undergone such intake with no apparent ill-effects (Klenner, 1971; Körner and Weber, 1972;* Hoffer, 1973; Poser, 1972). Further, other animals such as the gorilla ingest several grams daily. It is of course uncertain as to how far one can extrapolate from other animals to humans, and the concern— although probably applying to a very small proportion of the population—should not be ignored.

The point has been put to numerous individuals who have suffered greatly from respiratory malaises (such as nasal stuffiness and sinusitis) prior to mega vitamin C administration. Their almost invariable response (after two to three weeks administration when they found that it helped them considerably) has been that in view of the clear improvement/relief they have obtained while undergoing the mega vitamin intake, they would prefer to continue undergoing this administration rather than be subject to their previous miseries.

While taking due account of this concern as to possible unknown long-term adverse effects, it is also apposite to take the opposite standpoint that in view of the medical potential of mega vitamin C administration—as outlined in this monograph—it is more likely that individuals undergoing this administration are mostly much more likely to benefit from it than eventually to suffer from it.

---

* Korner and Weber (1972) considered numerous published clinical and experimental data. They concluded that generally there existed no indication of any effect prejudicial to health caused by vitamin C, even when administered in high doses; further, the frequency of slight gastrointestinal disturbances due to a laxative effect of the ascorbic acid (and in exceptional cases, allergic symptoms) was no greater than that of the signs of intolerance caused by other essential nutrients.

Chapter 8

Genetic aspects and biochemical individuality

8.1. Some aspects of utilization of ascorbate in relation to bio-chemical individuality*

The medical potential of mega vitamin C ingestion in many individuals is due to direct activity, AFR activity, and indirect activity via cyclic AMP, and is expressed in overall ability to buttress the defence mechanisms of the body. We have seen that elucidation of the extent of this potential is blurred by conditions in which the vitamin is destroyed or deactivated. Some of the variations in response to mega vitamin C administration can be classified under "biochemical individuality", by which is meant that the different responses in different individuals are due to variations in their physiology, past medical history and their eating habits, as well as to the effect of environmental conditions—or the interaction of environment and heredity—such as those encountered in environmental changes. Others appear to be inherent, as they seem to result from unalterable genetic characteristics. There exists, however, one other parameter which until recently has almost universally been considered to be non-existent, namely the variable ability of humans to biosynthesize ascorbate.

The important conclusion that humans are totally unable to biosynthesize vitamin C, and the elucidation of the daily levels of ascorbate requirements, are derived from medical information based mainly on Western or Western-oriented populations. It is relevant to stress that nomadic and desert tribes subsist on a diet composed primarily of cooked meat (such as that of the sheep); few, if any,

---

* The variation of ascorbate requirements in relation to biochemical individuality has been considered by Williams (1963) and Williams and Deason (1967) (see also Yew, 1974/5). Here we are concerned mainly at the molecular level.

174

fresh vegetables are consumed. The vitamin C content of such diets is very low indeed, and can be computed to be usually less than 2 mg daily. Yet scurvy manifestations have not been reported to be increased in these tribes.

In the days prior to the recognition of the role of vitamin C in the prevention of scurvy, a good proportion of sailors on long sea voyages succumbed to the disease. Yet some survived, and some were hardly affected by it. Thus, when Vasco de Gamma sailed round the Cape of Good Hope in 1498, one hundred of the crew of 160 men perished from the disease, but others survived (Harris, 1935). The individuals who suffered least from the disease must have had either

(i) A *very* low metabolic rate of ascorbate utilization;

(ii) decreased loss by deactivation (owing to a lower level of biosynthesis/activity of c-AMP PDE, and/or considerable ability to regenerate vitamin C from Del-A), or

(iii) ability to biosynthesize minimal quantities which can be expanded during absence of exogenous ascorbate.

Currently little is known concerning the factors which regulate the biosynthesis of PDE or which cause induction or potentiation of its activity apart from the requirement of c. neutral pH values for the optimum activity of most PDEs from different tissues and the requirement of one of the cations of Mg^{++}, Mn^{++}, Co^{++}, or Zn^{++}.* However, sufficient information is available for collation within the pattern that many humans are capable of some ascorbate biosynthesis, albeit well below the minimal daily requirements.

8.2. The potential of biosynthesis of ascorbate in humans

8.2.1. Comparison of *in vitro* results using tissue extracts with *in vivo* investigations in relation to the ascorbate balance sheet

Currently it is generally believed that humans, other primates, the guinea pig and several other species (see also section 5.1) are unable to biosynthesize vitamin C. This belief is based on *in vitro* and *in vivo* investigations. The *in vivo* investigations were concerned with the development of scurvy as a result of vitamin C deficient diets; the *in vitro* experiments utilized tissue homogenates in which the activity of the enzyme L-gulonolactone oxidase was assayed and found to be apparently absent (see Chapter 5). As a result of these and numerous

---

* Bourne *et al.* (1973) concluded that a c-AMP-dependent protein kinase is required for the regulation of synthesis of PDE.

other investigations (see section 5.3.1) the biosynthesis of ascorbate was found to form one arm of the ascorbate/xylulose fork. The overall scheme has already been presented in Fig. 5.2.

The apparent inability to biosynthesize ascorbate has been attributed to a "missing step" (Burns, 1957) involving the enzyme L-gulonolactone oxidase; Chatterjee *et al.* (1961) considered that there exists an additional missing step involving the enzyme glucuronolactonase. Other authors have attributed this defect specifically to "gene mutation" (Stone, 1966, 1972; Chatterjee *et al.*, 1975a).

A preliminary discussion has been given in section 5.4. Here we shall consider specifically the question whether there does exist any "missing step", or mutation in the biosynthesis sequence of ascorbate in man and other animals which appear unable to biosynthesize ascorbate.

In general, inability to demonstrate clearly the biosynthesis of ascorbate in tissue homogenates does not necessarily signify absence of a particular enzyme. The apparent defect could be due to the enzyme being deactivated by the products of the reactions or by an existing adverse factor. The latter may result from competition in the ascorbic biosynthetic fork, where despite an adequate activity of L-gulonolactone oxidase, ascorbate biosynthesis may be strongly inhibited by very high activities in formation of L-xylulose. This can be appreciated from Fig. 5.2.

The formation of H_2O_2 which accompanies the biosynthesis of 2-ketogulono-γ-lactone should be noted. H_2O_2 is likely to deactivate its parent enzyme L-gulono-γ-lactone oxidase, thereby tending to inhibit this step in ascorbate biosynthesis. This setback would normally be checked by the presence of catalase which decomposes H_2O_2. However, ascorbate in concentrations as low as 2×10^{-6} M inhibits the H_2O_2 decomposing activity of catalase (Orr, 1966, 1970). Hence, unless efficient compartmentalization exists, ascorbate formation would tend to inhibit its own biosynthesis. This facet applies also in respect of NADH, NAD, and NADPH activities since the parent nicotinamide forms a complex with ascorbate (see section 1.3.3.2).

Results of experiments *in vitro*, based on tissue homogenates, do not necessarily represent *in vivo* conditions. The latter conditions often rely on specific compartmentalizations, which may remove adverse products and may link thermodynamically improbable reactions to overwhelmingly spontaneous reactions, thereby enabling the originally improbable reactions to take place. Comparisons of data from tissue extracts with those from live animals—given in Table 8.1—support this contention.

Table 8.1. Comparison of percentage conversion data from *in vivo* experiments with those of *in vitro* experiments, using tissue extracts on the conversion of L-gulonolactone-1-C^{-4} to the corresponding L-ascorbic acid

Species	*In Vivo*	Liver tissue homogenates		Mitochondria
		Microsomes	Total homogenates	
Rat	9.1*	18.6†	12.0†	One quarter of the
	7.2*	10.0‡	8.0†§	activity of micro-
		7.7†‡§	3.6†	somes‡
		3.8†		
		7.7‖		
		26.1‖		
Guinea-pig	0.2*	0.05†	0.05†§	Stated to be "none"
	0.2*	0.05†‡§		but presumably < 0.2*
Monkey		0.07§		
Man		0.07§		

* Intraperitoneal injection of 12 mg L-gulonolactone-C^{14} (Burns and Evans, 1956).
† Burns *et al.* (1956).
‡ Burns (1967).
§ Burns *et al.* (1957).
‖ Hassan and Lehninger using a tissue homogenate medium enriched with ATP, DPN, Mg^{++} and nicotinamide (Hassan and Lehninger, 1956).

The data in Table 8.1 give rise to several suggestions:

Mitochondrial participation in ascorbate biosynthesis. Rat liver mitochondria display about a quarter of the activity of microsomes in the conversion of L-gulonolactone oxidase to L-ascorbic acid (Burns *et al.*, 1956). The findings of Hassan and Lehninger (1956) that enrichment of tissue homogenates with ATP, nicotinamide and other substances improved ascorbate biosynthesis, and the somewhat higher percentage conversion values in live guinea-pigs as compared to their tissue extracts—suggest that extrapolation from *in vitro* and *in vivo* conditions in regard to total inability to biosynthesize ascorbate in guinea-pigs (and in man) is not valid.

Chatterjee *et al.* (1961) considered that the biosynthetic contribution of mitochondria could have been due to some adhering microsomes despite three washings. However, this conclusion should be contrasted with the findings by Kersten *et al.* (1956) that despite numerous washings mitochondria from pigs adrenals still contained 30 mg ascorbate per 100 mg dry weight.

Interference with biosynthetic routes. Homogenization and centrifugation in sucrose gradients could adversely affect L-ascorbate biosynthesis by interfering with the original balance and sequence in the biosynthetic paths following decreased extent of compartmentalization. A thorough comparison of biosynthesis of ascorbate using *tissue slices* with those employing extracts in evaluating activity of L-gulonolactone oxidase is desirable but does not appear to have taken place.

Unaccounted ascorbic acid. The percentage conversion data given in Table 8.1 did not allow for the ability of phosphodiesterase to hydrolyse effectively the lactone structure of ascorbate (see section 3.3.2) and for the formation of L-2-ascorbate sulphate from ascorbate (Baker *et al.*, 1971); these reactions were not known at the time. It has been computed that as much as 30 to 50 mg L-ascorbate-2-sulphate are produced daily in man (Baker *et al.*, recorded by Sauberlich *et al.*, 1975), and also that some is excreted in the faeces (Hornig, 1974). When allowance is made for the daily production of both compounds and the relevant half-life time of ascorbate of *c*. 16 to 28 days (Atkins *et al.*, 1964; Hellman and Burns, 1958; Baker *et al.*, 1962) the total quantity of products of ascorbic acid—expressed in terms of equivalent ascorbic acid—is likely to exceed significantly the amount of ingested ascorbate, thereby indicating that some ascorbate must be endogenous in man, and possibly in other animals, considered to be "deficient" in vitamin C biosynthesis. Such men (or animals) although capable of ascorbate biosynthesis (to a level falling short of that required to prevent scurvy in non-stressed conditions) are clearly not able to raise their output to the increased requirements in stress-conditions. Animals which do not respond by increased biosynthesis of ascorbate are bound therefore to display correspondingly pronounced malfunctions; the defect can be rectified by exogenous supply of ascorbate-rich diet. This approach is supported by the genetic considerations and observations of enzyme synthesis in mammals as well as by evidence obtained directly from humans.

During embryonic development various genes of any given species (and therefore of a specific DNA) are partly or wholly suppressed, or activated, resulting in the development of different tissues and associated respective enzyme suppression or activity (for numerous references, see Schjeide and De Vellis, 1970).

Three classes of observation are relevant to the thesis that the apparent inability to biosynthesize ascorbate is due to mutation or deletion of the gene(s) responsible for L-gulonolactone oxidase (and aldonolactone oxidase).

De Fabro (1967) established that there exists a significant activity of L-gulonolactone oxidase in the embryos of guinea-pigs in contrast with disappearance of this activity in adult guinea-pigs. The only possible explanation is that the gene responsible for L-gulonolactone oxidase does form part of the genome of guinea-pigs, but that its expression is suppressed partly or wholly in the adult by regulatory proteins, or that the activity is not apparent because the competitive activity of the enzymes in the L-xylulose part of the biosynthetic fork is overwhelmingly greater in the adult.

The findings of Yew (1975) and Chatterjee *et al*. (1975) are in accord with this interpretation. Yew (1975) found that ascorbic acid concentrations in embryonic tissues differed distinctly from those in post-embryonic tissues, and concluded that ascorbic acid bio-synthesis may take place in rapidly differentiating guinea-pig embryonic brain cells. Chatterjee *et al*. (1975) observed that *in vivo* L-gulonolactone oxidase activity is affected by hydrocortisone and by insulin at the level of enzyme synthesis.

Baker *et al*. (1960) demonstrated that healthy humans who were given D-glucuronolactone excreted excess ascorbate, but did not do so when they were fed with D-glucuronic acid. Subsequently, Baker *et al*. (1962) demonstrated that about one quarter of D-glucurono-lactone-6-C^{14} fed to healthy men and women was converted to L-ascorbate. It is relevant that the first group of investigators examined both plasma and urine, while the second group assayed the urine only. In view of the length of the half-life time of ascorbate in humans, some of the ascorbate formed must be retained in tissues such as the adrenals, pituitary and leucocytes in addition to those noted in urine and plasma. Further, some of the ascorbate present in the body undergoes a change to L-ascorbate-2-sulphate, some of which is excreted in the faeces (Hornig, 1974), and about 30 to 60 mg daily in the urine, both of which effects were unknown in the early sixties. Also some of the ascorbate is delactonized. The percentage of conversion of L-glucuronolactone to L-ascorbate itself can therefore reasonably be corrected to a proportion significantly higher than a quarter.*

The capacity of microsomal fractions containing L-gulonolactone-oxidase from the livers of mammals established as ascorbate synthe-sizers varies significantly. In terms of mg ascorbate synthesized

---

* It is worthwhile pondering that the quantity of vitamin C biosynthesized in humans could be drastically reduced by hydrolytic delactonization if the PDE was insufficiently separated from the sites of the biosynthesis. This possibility cannot be dismissed out of hand since Cheung and Salganicoff (1967) observed substantial latent PDE activity in a microsomal fraction of the nerve endings of rat brain cerebra.

(μg/mg protein/hour) the variation is from maximum in the goat
(~68), cow (~50), rat (~38), rabbit (~26) to a minimum in the cat
and dog (~5); see Chatterjee (1973). As these variations were
obtained using identical experimental conditions, the decreased
activity must be due to decreased formation of L-gulonolactone
oxidase biosynthesized in the various animals. The variation can be
understood readily in terms of increased suppression of the structural
gene activities by the corresponding regulatory proteins (see also
section 5.4).

8.2.2. Genetic origins of biochemical individuality

Genetic diversity in the human population ensures variation
between individuals in their capacity to undertake biochemical
reactions. Some diversity may exist as a polymorphism, that is it is
stably maintained in the population, while other diversity may be
transient in the sense that it is the subject of a progressing
evolutionary change. Although it is clear that, as the result of
evolutionary change, humans have a much reduced ability to biosynthesize ascorbate compared with other mammals, variations due
to genetic differences mean that the extent of this ability should
display biochemical individuality.

At the molecular level, the source of this genetic variation may lie
with either of two cellular locations of genetic material. The DNA of
the nucleus is believed to be invariant in sequence throughout all the
cells of a given animal; however, it is not established whether all
mitochondria within a given tissue contain the same DNA sequence
or even whether all the mitochondria within the same cell are
identical. In addition to variation between individuals, it is therefore
possible that there might be variation within the mitochondria of an
individual. We might further note that in fertilization the sperma-
tozoal mitochondria are lost when the mid sheath or tail to which
they are attached is left behind and does not enter the ovum;
mitochondria are therefore maternal in origin. Some of the variation
in ability to biosynthesize ascorbate may be mitochondrial in origin
(and see section 9.3.4).

8.2.3. Conclusions

We may sum up by concluding that the available experimental
data on ascorbate biosynthesis—or apparent lack of it—may be

interpreted within a conceptual framework in which animals requiring exogenous ascorbate still possess the gene sequences required for the biosynthesis of L-glucuronolactonase, L-glucurono-reductase and L-gulono-lactone-oxidase, and do indeed biosynthesize them. However, L-gulono-lactonase is overwhelmingly active in the displacement of the equilibrium towards L-gulonic acid, and/or L-gulonic-dehydrogenase is also overwhelmingly active in the formation of 3-keto-gulonic acid, thereby reducing ascorbate biosynthesis below the minimal requirements. On this basis the concepts of a "missing step" or of mutation involving evolutionary deletion of L-gulono-lactone-oxidase are not tenable. Indeed, the failure of a species to biosynthesize a particular substance need not result from gene deletion, but can be explained in terms of changes in regulatory functions.

8.3. Ascorbate requirements in individuals in relation to associated hydrolytic delactonization by PDE and to other parameters (see also section 7.4)

Preliminary experiments we have carried out *in vitro* indicate that under otherwise apparently identical experimental conditions PDEs from different sources can vary considerably in their abilities to hydrolyse ascorbate (see section 3.3.2). Such variation may depend in part on the respective concentration ratios of the high affinity and low affinity forms of PDE and on respective particulate and non-particulate activities.

In vivo the situation is complicated by the competition of c-AMP and ascorbate for association with PDE, and by the rate of transfer of ascorbate across the various membranes of different tissue cells. The higher the c-AMP concentration levels the less ascorbate will be competitively associated and hydrolysed by PDE and vice versa. The rate of utilization of ascorbate can therefore vary considerably with the individual and with the stress conditions to which he is being subjected.

Calculations comprising every single parameter in the utilization and loss of ascorbate can be very tedious. There is however no need to go into detail; the approximate limits of the ranges covering most individuals can be arrived at on the following simplified basis.

The concentrations of c-AMP in the tissues vary during the day and are subject to different conditions such as those of ATP availability, adenylcyclase activity and PDE activity. From a survey of the vast literature available it can be computed that variations to a maximum of a hundred-fold can take place. A hundred-fold decrease in c-AMP levels can—in the region of competitive concentrations—be associated with a hundred-fold increase in ascorbate association and its hydrolysis by PDE. Additional factors which can affect the daily intake of vitamin C are (i) oxidation and delactonization prior to absorption into the blood (a factor of c. up to ten-fold); (ii) renal threshold variation from c. 1.2 to 1.8 mg per 100 ml blood; (iii) small variations in sulphation of ascorbate, and (iv) transformation into xylulose excreted in pentosuria.

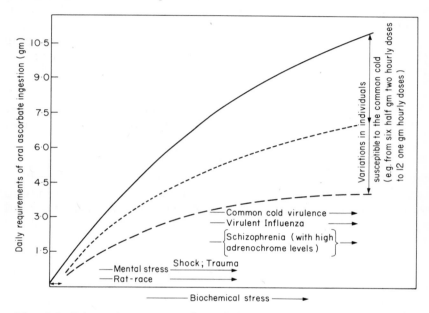

Fig. 8.1. Schematic representation of the feasible variations of vitamin C total daily therapeutic administration, with biochemical stress.

In general the probability of a parameter $A(P_A)$ dependent on two different parameters B and C is a function of the product of their respective magnitudes, thus

$$P_A \; \alpha \; (P_B \times P_C).$$

It follows that the variation in vitamin C requirements by different individuals allowing for the various parameters noted, is of the order of a hundred- to a thousand-fold. If the "minimal" ideal antiscurvy-based requirement of ascorbate are in the region of 5 to 20 mg daily, the *probability range* for the needs of ascorbate extended by a hundred-fold to a thousand-fold is between 0.5 to 20 g. However, if the probability of oxidation and delactonization prior to absorption into the blood is eliminated, the range is likely to lie between the very approximate limits of 0.2 to 10 g daily. The variations can be represented arbitrarily as in Fig. 8.1.

Chapter 9

Overall view: Present problems and future developments

9.1. Overview of biosynthesis, dosage and evolutionary aspects of ascorbic acid

The medical potential of vitamin C is known to be expressed in various fields such as the inhibition of scurvy, the formation of collagen, and general repair of wounds and damaged tissues. For unstressed activities such as minor scratches, it would appear that quantities in the region of 70 to 150 mg daily (which vary with the conclusions of different investigators) may be sufficient to meet the requirements of many individuals. However, modern life gives rise to ever-greater extents of biochemical stress conditions with correspondingly overall higher levels of activities such as increased biosynthesis of neurohormones, increased requirements for antibodies and increased anti-histamine control, malfunctions following decreased cyclic AMP levels, and decreased resistance to malaises. The resultant additional requirements/malfunctions can be satisfied/corrected by corresponding ascorbate availability which in turn can be met only by higher intake of ascorbic acid. This must be raised to still higher levels because of irreversible oxidative degradation and deactivation by delactonization of the vitamin arising from oral administration. A further loss arises because the proportion of absorbed ascorbate decreases with the increased level of the dose following intervention of the renal threshold. This makes it rather difficult to compute the precise oral ingestion requirements of vitamin C prophylaxis under modern biochemical stress conditions; nevertheless it is possible to conclude that in many individuals, if not most, the indications are that the optimum dosage required is several times larger than that which is at present strongly defended by the orthodox Establishment.

The practical limit of the individual vitamin C dose taken by different persons does vary. My investigations have shown that some individuals can take 2 g in a single dose without experiencing any discomfort. Others suffer gastrointestinal discomfort when each dose exceeds 0.4 to 0.6 g. A few are subject to flushing of the face when they exceed 0.3 g. Hence the limit of each dose has to be determined by the particular individual.

It is worthwhile stressing that although most humans follow well-defined *patterns* of physiological and biochemical activities, not all of them follow precisely the same network of metabolic activities, since the mechanisms and efficiencies of homeostatic controls can differ significantly from one group of individuals to another when they differ genetically, in their eating habits and in exposure to different environmental conditions.

Genetically, many individuals are likely to biosynthesize ascorbate, although to different extents many of which are well below the minimal daily vitamin C requirements. In some the homeostatic controls may be such that the extra ascorbate required to overcome the effects of biochemical stress may be minimal. In certain cases however mega vitamin C therapy, such as the administration of 1 g every hour for the first eight to ten hours, is essential to overcome the onslaught of the common cold.

The ingestion of ascorbate must be undertaken under conditions minimizing its deactivation and its destruction as well as under conditions minimizing the gastrointestinal discomfort to which some individuals are prone.

9.2. Differences in the rationales of different schools for mega administration

The minimal daily requirements of vitamin C computed by different investigators were based on the limits of incidence of scurvy plus a small margin. These requirements apply primarily to unstressed individuals who are not susceptible to respiratory and other malaises. In view of biochemical individuality these allowances cannot be accepted as the limit or even as a guide in the case of biochemically stressed individuals where the overactivity of histamine and overactivity of PDE can be corrected pharmacologically by the use of mega administration of the vitamin.

It is apposite to stress the difference between the standpoint of the usefulness of mega intake advanced here and those of Pauling and Stone. Pauling bases his recommendations on mega vitamin C administration on the amounts of the vitamin in diets consumed by primates and other animals which are believed not to be able to biosynthesize ascorbic acid, and on the amounts biosynthesized by animals capable of the biosynthesis. He extrapolates in terms of dose/kg weight to the human. In the circumstances this type of extrapolation is inescapable. However, since the physiology, metabolism and genetics of the animals are not strictly comparable to man, it can be argued that there must be some uncertainty as to the accuracy of the extrapolation.

Stone (1972) backs his advocacy by the arguments that our early ancestors were likely to have biosynthesized multigram quantities of vitamin C daily. He considers that as a result of (a *presumed*) gene deletion millions of years ago, the later ancestors of man, primates and other animals lost the ability to biosynthesize the vitamin. However, in view of the considerations advanced in Chapter 8, such deletion and mutation need not necessarily have taken place.

The considerations presented here are based on a different conceptual framework, namely that the usefulness of mega administration of the vitamin is to be found partly in the intrinsic needs in humans which can rise multifold with the need for body repairs such as those involving increased collagen formation and antibody formation. A separate factor is the ability of ascorbate at *high* concentrations to act as an inhibitor of PDE (as well as assisting at one stage in the sequence of events leading to c-AMP formation) and thereby to retard the hydrolysis of c-AMP and c-GMP. The considerable increase in stress and strain to which humans are exposed in this technological age favours depressed c-GMP levels, thereby upsetting minimal physiological requirements. Raising the tissues' ascorbate levels above the "normal" levels (of *c.* 1–1.4 mg/100 ml plasma) resists these depressions and even raises them somewhat. The physiological results of pharmacological administration of mega ascorbate, while most helpful, can hardly be considered a truly "vitamin-activity" because of the size of the dose. Further, the size of the dose required increases with the losses encountered as a result of the method used in administration of the "vitamin".

9.3. Possible approaches to correction of the deficiency in bio-synthesis of ascorbate in humans

9.3.1. Desirable criteria of approaches to correction of the deficiency

Currently, approaches to correction of the deficiency of ascorbate biosynthesis in humans are based upon the provision of diets with high ascorbate content or by oral ingestion. However, it is worth-while considering other ways in which the deficiency could be overcome. Any proposed method should

  (i) be capable of uncomplicated withdrawal, or ready modifi-cation or correction in the light of future developments, and
  (ii) cause negligible interference with other physiological mechan-isms, unless specifically desired.

Several approaches which can satisfy these limitations can be visualized such as (i) the use of diets enhancing vitamin C bio-synthesis, (ii) introduction of bacteria capable of vitamin C bio-synthesis into the alimentary canal, and (iii) changes in existing genetic control and suppression of ascorbate biosynthesis.

Currently, little is known concerning the potential of these approaches. Nevertheless, these possibilities deserve some examin-ation and will therefore be considered in turn.

9.3.2. Diets enhancing biosynthesis of ascorbate*

A significant amount of information is available in respect of enzyme induction in bacteria and other procaryotes. However, extrapolation from this field to one involving humans is likely to be hedged by so many ifs and buts that it is unlikely to be practical. Extrapolation to humans is more feasible from researches on our close relations, such as chimpanzees or baboons. Any researches should comprise assays of ascorbate in leucocytes, plasma and urine; parallel c-AMP evaluations should be included.

9.3.3. Introduction into the gut of bacterial mutants capable of biosynthesizing ascorbate

At present, the potential of the alimentary canal as a host to useful bacteria does not appear to have been sufficiently explored or exploited in practice. There has not been a search for bacteria biosynthesizing ascorbate effectively. However, in view of the enor-mous number of available and potential mutants it should not be an impossible task to find and develop such bacteria, some variety of which could exist in the alimentary canal alone or supported by other bacteria. The elimination of intestinal bacteria by the use of antibiotics is well known and should be undertaken first. The

---

* It is interesting that Svirbely (1936) concluded that adequate supply of the vitamin B complex is essential for obtaining normal vitamin C values in certain tissues of the rat. Sasmal et al. (1968) reported that both manganese and cobalt stimulated the synthesis of L-ascorbic acid from L-gulonolactone, in rats.

bacteria could then orally be introduced into the bacteria-freed alimentary canal in special capsules which would be time released to pass the pyloric sphincter into the duodenum or further on as necessary.

9.3.4. Changes in existing genetic control of ascorbate biosynthesis using mitochondria

Biochemical genetics can be manipulated by incorporation into, or deletion of, existing genes from the genetic template. Such incorporation or deletion is carried out nowadays in bacterial and viral genomes. The incorporation or deletion of genes in the DNA complex of eucaryotes is known to take place, e.g. the incorporation of genes from herpes virus into the human genome. However, the technique of manipulation of such changes in the DNA of eucaryotes has so far not been developed anywhere near the level practised in bacteria and viruses.

The genetic templates of humans and primates (and other animals lower in the evolutionary sequence) comprise DNAs in the nucleus, in the nucleolus and in the mitochondrion. One possible approach towards manipulation of the genetic constitution of eucaryotes may be via their mitochondria, a point that is relevant to considering changes in the ability to biosynthesize ascorbate.

Mitochondria are known to cooperate metabolically with nuclear DNAs by utilizing proteins whose biosynthesis is coded for by the nuclear DNA; also some of the twenty-five or thirty proteins coded for by the mitochondrial DNA are considered capable of participation in exo-mitochondrial activities. All mitochondria in a given species or in the same tissue are not necessarily identical; immunological differences are known to exist between male mitochondria and female mitochondria. Mitochondrial inheritance is maternal. Further, during cell division there is no certainty that the mitochondria are equally divided between the two daughter cells.

Plant mitochondria are known to be involved in biosynthesis of ascorbate. It has been already noted in section 5.4 that in the rat mitochondria do contribute to ascorbate biosynthesis, albeit to a quarter of the total synthesis.

Mitochondria are usually considered to be self-replicating, and thus likely to retain the characteristics of the female parent. The feasibility of biochemical genetics using mitochondria deserves careful consideration. Selection of mitochondria or their manipulation to form specific mutants with pronounced abilities to biosynthesize ascorbate—although not a short-term research project—is by no means an unlikely attainment. It does of course involve a number of practical problems which will have to be solved. However, the potential of genetic manipulation by utilizing them introduces another dimension to biochemical engineering.

9.4. Considerations relating to other future investigations

9.4.1. Biosynthesis of ascorbate

It is difficult to evaluate the intrinsic potential of endogenous ascorbate biosynthesis. It is quite possible that the level of ascorbate biosynthesis in humans is considerably affected by the dietary protein control, the dietary supplementation of particular metal ions, and the physiological hormone balance. This possibility is supported by the results of Chatterjee *et al.* (1975) who, in their investigations in animals, showed that L-gulonolactone oxidase activity is very strikingly altered in application of such conditions.

These and the previous considerations (see Chapter 8) open a new field of research into the possibility of control of ascorbate biosynthesis in humans. However, before undertaking such researches it is essential to consider the phrasing of the overall problem. It is not sufficient to ask simply whether ascorbate is biosynthesized or not; or whether L-gulonolactone oxidase (and other enzymes of the ascorbate pathway) are biosynthesized or not. From the considerations given in section 8.2 it should be clear that there is unlikely to have been any "missing step" or "gene-mutation" or "gene-deletion". The deficiency in ascorbate biosynthesis is evidently not a case of *permanent* suppression of enzyme biosynthesis, since the embryos of guinea pigs have been shown to exert L-gulonolactone oxidase activity. It seems to be a case in which *regulatory proteins* involved in activation/suppression of the structural genes concerned have allowed/enforced gene activation at the embryo stage only to follow this by subsequent suppression. The problem is therefore what causes gene suppression to take place and whether it is economically wise or physiologically useful to reverse it. The use of some tissue extracts may seem inescapable, but the conclusions drawn from such experiments where the biologically-enforced compartmentalization has been eliminated makes extrapolation uncertain. Of necessity, research will involve the use of live animals, some of which must be as nearly related as possible to humans. Chimpanzees, which also require exogenous ascorbic acid, appear to offer a very near substitute. As a species they are very close to humans. Their percentage sequence difference in DNA (compared with humans) has been computed to be only 1.1% (e.g. King and Wilson, 1975). This signifies that a strand of human DNA which is *c*. 3000 nucleotides long (and which therefore can code for a sequence of 1000 amino acids in protein/enzymes) can be differentiated from the equivalent chimpanzee strand at about 33 sites only. Currently, this difference is the smallest attainable in searching for a substitute for humans.

9.4.2. Contribution of PDE and AFR

Having accepted the concept that the effect of rise in ascorbate presence results in increased probability of AFR activities (in aerated conditions, and in conditions where linking to ascorbic oxidase activity is a practical possibility) and in the inhibition of phosphodiesterase activity, future investigations are likely to be more profitable if both these factors are taken into consideration. It is clear that the number of problems to be tackled is large. Further, their elucidation requires clarity in differentiation between cause and effect or symptoms; otherwise invalid conclusions may be arrived at.

As an example consider the problem of ageing: Since c-AMP and c-GMP affect numerous biological activities, the question may well be posed whether there is a relationship between the lowering of c-AMP levels and c-GMP levels and ageing. If there is—and the indications are that this is likely to be so—at least in a proportion of the population—it would be natural to pose the question: How far and how long can we utilize increased ascorbate levels to control PDE activity and/or high AFR levels? However, to increase the probability of obtaining meaningful answers in such investigations we have to probe first the question of cause and effect, namely: Does the overall process of ageing cause or involve an overall increase in PDE activity as a result of which c-AMP levels decrease? Or is the process of ageing a result of decreased c-AMP levels? Or is the process of ageing merely paralleled by changes in PDE activity?

Further, before we can embark on the above investigations we have to answer other fundamental questions regarding the mechanism of PDE activity and the possibility of its variation in different tissues.

Variable activities of PDE from different sources. For the sake of convenience, PDE was considered as a single entity in the previous discussions. However, it is known that a number of variants do exist. Thus there are in the rat liver two recognized types of PDE, namely the high affinity (higher Km value) and the lower affinity (lower Km value) forms (e.g. Brooker *et al.*, 1968). PDE from different tissues have different Km values (for several references and Table see Cheung, 1970). It has been found in both particulate and soluble fractions, see Appleman *et al.* (1973) and it has been suggested that it is an allosteric enzyme. Tisdale (1975) reported that both AA and DHA are reversible inhibitors of both high and low affinity forms of PDE from Walker carcinoma whereas only the high affinity form of the enzyme from rat liver was inhibited by DHA.

Such variations indicate that PDEs from different tissues can differ to extents that can be reflected not only in capacity for ascorbate inhibition but possibly even in ability to hydrolyse the lactone structure of the vitamin. This approach can explain the differences between the percentage inhibitions noted by Moffat and Owen (1972), by the author, and by Buck and Zadunaisky (1975). However, the reaction media and the procedures also differed with the investigators and this would be an additional and possibly a preponderant factor. Certainly the older the ascorbate solution and the older the PDE solution (although kept strictly refrigerated) the greater the difference in percentage inhibition. Further our investigations were carried out under strict anaerobic conditions and in the almost total absence of light, whereas these precautions do not appear to have been enforced by the other investigators.

The effect of the ascorbic system on c-AMP levels has been considered previously in terms of competitive ascorbate interaction only. However, it can be computed that the ascorbate free radical and DHA (particularly in the hydrated anionic form) should be capable of inhibiting PDE. In this monograph evidence has been presented that ascorbate interacts with PDE: evidence for the interaction of AFR^- with PDE is as yet unavailable but evidence that DHA inhibits only the high affinity form of PDE has been reported by Tisdale (1975). What is not known as yet is whether DHA is hydrolysed by PDE as ascorbate is. If so, this would represent an additional irreversible path by which ascorbate levels are reduced, since DHA is capable of being reversibly reduced to ascorbate while the hydrolysed product 2:3-diketoglutonic acid is not (see also Fig. 1.4).

Influence of c-AMP. The inductive effect of cyclic AMP at the transcription level on the biosynthesis of a number of enzymes raises

the possibility that a number of other enzymes—so far not investigated—may also prove to be induced at the transcription level by
this nucleotide. Three associated questions naturally arise:

  (i) What are the respective c-AMP levels at which various enzym-
      atic inductions take place? Could there be a *sequence* of
      specific activations associated with increasing c-AMP levels?

 (ii) Are such controls likely to be located only at the transcrip-
      tion level?

(iii) Since cyclic AMP formation takes place in the cytoplasm or
      at the cell membrane (when the adenylcyclase activity is
      particulate only) what controls the rate of entry of c-AMP
      into the nucleus? Are there threshold limits?

Ascorbate has been shown to be present in nuclei of calf thymus
(Stern and Timmonen, 1954); and in wheat nuclei it was shown
capable of replacing glutathione in m-RNA synthesis (Price, 1966). If
c-AMP formation is restricted to the cytoplasm, then the significance of the potential of ascorbate when in the nucleus is likely to
involve other activities than maintenance of c-AMP levels.

The potential of ascorbate in retarding of ageing is not yet clearly
defined. Excessive free radical formation of various biological free
radicals has been implicated in the ageing process; and it has been
suggested that AFR can retard ageing by scavenging the undesirable
free radical in biological organizations. The anti-oxidant activity of
ascorbate, which can be expressed also in its free radical state, has
also been implicated in the anti-ageing trend (e.g. Tappel, 1968;
Comfort *et al.*, 1971). Ageing could also be due to slowing down or
suppression of activity of regulatory proteins because of reduced
c-AMP levels which are no longer within the range required to
activate their formation. If this be the case, increased ascorbate levels
can perform a most useful service in maintaining c-AMP levels
without subjecting humans to unacceptable levels of toxicity.

9.4.3. Ascorbate inhibition of herpes-virus development in relation to possible virus participation in carcinogenesis

Herpes HSV-2 has been considered to be implicated in carcinogenesis (for references see Hausen, 1975). Recently observations have
been made which have been interpreted as indicating that HSV-1 is
also a candidate for precipitation in carcinogenesis (Tarro and
Hollingshead, 1973). As yet there appears to be no evidence that the
genitally located HSV-2 is susceptible to deactivation by sufficiently
high ascorbate concentrations; but there is considerable evidence that

the orally sited HSV-1 is inhibited effectively by high ascorbate intake (see section 7.7.3).

Three major questions require appropriate investigations and answers:

  (i) How far can ascorbate treatment inhibit development of HSV-2?

 (ii) What is the mechanism of inhibition of HSV-1 by ascorbate; does the inhibition extend to inhibition of any potential participation in carcinogenesis?

(iii) The concept that virus latency is due to integration of an appropriate section of the virus in the human genome is generally regarded as reasonable. Since maintenance of high ascorbate levels appears a pre-requisite, does this signify that the "products" of the virus section integrated in the human genome are being "neutralized" in some way? Or is the inhibition due to the blocking of a subsequent stage?

It is apposite to point out that cyclic AMP has been shown to inhibit tumour development (see section 7.7.6.6). It is worthwhile therefore to consider whether ascorbate may act directly via AFR and/or via cyclic AMP to inhibit carcinogenesis by these herpes viruses.

9.4.4 Considerations relating to a combined administration of magnesium and ascorbate in the treatment of conditions associated with calcification and fatty deposition

9.4.4.1. *Overview*

It has already been emphasized that mega ascorbic intake should not be regarded as a universal panacea for all ailments. It is also necessary to stress that its use need not result in maximum benefits because the symptoms being treated may well arise from either an ascorbate-independent activity or from a combination of causes in which ascorbate can affect only one of the factors concerned or because of aggravating complications. Atherosclerosis can be used in illustration of possible difficulties.

This pathological condition is associated with diseases of the coronary and cerebral arteries. There exist lesions (plaques) with high cholesterol content sited in subendothelial stratum of the arterial intima. The disease progresses as the cholesterol accumulates in the form of fluid or crystals in the phagocytes which collect at these sites; and following this, connective tissue proliferates. Deeper strata of the intima are then invaded and necrosis takes place as the connective tissues lack sufficient nourishment (as a result of inhibition of plasma diffusion). Later on calcification takes place (see also sections 7.7.5.1 to 7.7.5.3).

Depending on the age of the disease, amelioration and reversal require decalcification as well as de-cholesterolization, and formation of new collagen in the process of regeneration of the tissues. Whereas de-cholesterolization is likely to be achieved by significant increases in cholesterol metabolism (which can be enhanced by ascorbate affecting c-AMP levels), de-calcification is likely to be enhanced by magnesium being exchanged for calcium. Further, decreased trends for the process of calcification are likely to be favoured by increasing the $\{[Mg^{++}]/[Ca^{++}]\}$ ratio in administration or in particular foods, or in hard-water districts where the water contains significant quantities of magnesium. It is therefore to be expected that the incidence of vascular coronary disease should be lower in hard-water districts. However, it should be borne in mind that much of the water drunk in hard-water areas is in the form of tea, coffee or cocoa which is initially boiled. The process of boiling removes most of the magnesium (and calcium) as carbonates, and thus this source of magnesium is much depleted. It is probably for this reason that the available statistical evidence obtained (for references see Bloch, 1973) shows only part of the potential trend.

The entry of Ca^{++} into the muscle is required in muscular contraction (which accompanies shortening of the sarcomere—i.e. between the thin and thick filaments of muscle) whereas absence of Ca^{++} favours maintenance of the cross-bridges in the relaxed form of the muscle. The muscular activities are mediated by ATP $\underset{}{\overset{hydrolysis}{\rightleftharpoons}}$ ADP + Pi formation and reformation which require the enzyme ATPase the activity of which is associated with Mg^{++}. The balance of activities could clearly be affected by excessive availability of Ca^{++} (which would favour prolongation of muscular contraction) and by smaller availability of Mg^{++} (which would tend to retard ATPase activity). Hence contributions to the maintenance of the physiologically correct ratio of $\{[Ca^{++}]/[Mg^{++}]\}$ is not only desirable, but is essential.

In common with other physiological concentration ratios, this ratio could vary within a narrow range; however, at the end and over this latitude, higher ratios would favour a longer period of muscular contraction, and vice versa. Maintenance of the physiological levels of the ratio is attained by a number of factors. The parathyroid hormone is known to be sensitive to serum Ca^{++} and to be involved in Ca^{++} transport across membranes and in the release of Ca^{++} from mitochondria; it would therefore be expected to exercise some control over the range of $\{[Ca^{++}]/[Mg^{++}]\}$.* Diet can reasonably be expected to contribute to the trends affecting the ratio. High Ca-content foods and comparatively less Mg comprising high-protein content, such as milk and cheese, would favour Ca^{++} levels. Further, Ca^{++} and Mg^{++} concentration levels are interdependent, as it is known that increased magnesium intake is accompanied by increased calcium excretion in the faeces and in the urine.

The calcification potential is generally greater in individuals with diets rich in protein and calcium but comparatively deficient in magnesium. Most of the calcium and magnesium ingested in absence of chelating agents is precipitated as phosphate (or carbonate) in the intestines. A protein-rich diet provides a high content of peptides/ amino acids (in the intestines) which chelate multivalent cations present thereby keeping them in solution and enhancing their absorption via the intestinal wall into blood/lymph. Thus, milk, cheese and other dairy products which are rich in calcium and comparatively poorer in magnesium increase the probability of calcification.

A magnesium/ascorbate administration should aid in lowering the trends for calcification and also relevant withdrawal of lipids from the plaques. It is apposite to stress that on ageing, individuals exposed to conditions favouring the formation of Ca/phospholipid/ cholesterol plaques tend to form more, larger and stabler plaques, thereby making their dispersal increasingly more difficult and consequently aggravating the condition. It is relevant that Anitschkow (1933) noted that (following cholesterol withdrawal from the diet) gradual disappearance of lipid from large plaques in rabbits could take as much as two to three years. Considering the relative life span of rabbits and humans, it may be that total resorption of the plaques may not be obtained in the more aged individuals; nevertheless the trends favouring increased manifestation of these conditions could be strongly inhibited.

9.4.4.3. Dosage

The daily ascorbic dose should comprise three times daily each about 1 g. The magnesium can be conveniently taken as magnesium

---

* Both Ca^{++} and cyclic AMP are involved in the action of parathyroid hormone on embryonic bone *in vitro* (Hermann-Erlee *et al.*, 1975).

hydroxide, and should be about 0.15 g three times daily. Larger doses of magnesium hydroxide (e.g. 0.3 to 0.6 g a single dose can be taken by individuals suffering from acidity; however over-dosage of acid-neutralizing substances should be avoided so as not to induce development of alkalosis. Magnesium citrate can be taken in some-what larger equivalent doses, but this salt is not available usually in B.P. or equivalent grades.

It must be emphasized that the magnesium/ascorbate should be administered with protein meals—for the reasons given. One con-venient way is to take one of the doses with warm milk (flavoured with cocoa or other suitable additives) before sleep.

9.4.4.4. *Types of trials*

The use of placebo and double-blind trials is generally considered essential; yet they introduce their own uncertainties, see the first and second footnotes on section 7.7.2.1.

It is apposite to stress that allowance should be made for numerous variables such as the effects on participants of:

    (i)   Stresses subjected to in the course of one's environment;
   (ii) body parameters such as overweight and oedoema;
 (iii) diet and quantity of liquids drunk daily;
 (iv) excesses undergone in various activities such as alcohol intake (or other drugs), food intake and sexual intercourse;
  (v) age and sex, and
 (vi) amount of exercise taken daily.

Enforcement of placebo and double-blind trials can be unproductive unless strict attention is paid to the different involvements of the various participants.

Many more problems can be raised and, indeed, have to be tackled. One remembers the words of Chargaff when reviewing the newly developed concept of the DNA double helix: "We have put a ladder into the heavens, but a hundred years or more will elapse before we have mounted the first rung". Let us hope that in a very much shorter time many of the problems facing us will have been solved.

References

A

Abbasy, M. A. (1937). The diuretic action of vitamin C. *Biochem. J.* **31**, 339-342.

Abdulla, Y. H. and Hamadah, K. (1970). 3',5'-cyclic adenosine monophosphate in depression and mania. *Lancet* (21 Feb.), 378-381.

Abderhalden, E. (1937). Weitere Beobachtungen uber die Einwirkung von Ascorbinsäure (Vitamin C) auf Aminosaüren. *Fermentforschung* **15**, 360-381.

Abt, A. F., Von Schuching, S., Enns, T. (1963) Vitamin C requirements of man re-examined. *Amer. J. Clin. Nutrition* **12**, 21-29.

Ackerfeldt, S. (1957). Oxidation of N-N-dimethyl-p-phenylenediamine by serum from patients with mental disease. *Science* **125**, 117-119.

Allen, M. J., Boyland, E., Dukes, C. E., Horning, E. S. and Watson, G. J. (1957). Cancer of the urinary bladder induced in mice with metabolites of aromatic amines and tryptophan. *Brit. J. Cancer* **11**, 212-228.

Anderson, J., Grande, F. and Keys, A. (1958). Dietary ascorbic acid and serum cholesterol. *Fed. Proceed.* **17**, 468.

Anderson, B. M., Reid, D. B. W. and Beaton, G. H. (1972). Vitamin C and the common cold: A double-blind trial. *Can. Med. A. J.* **107**, 503-508.

Anderson, T. W., Suranyi, G. and Beaton, G. H. (1974). The effect on winter illness of large doses of vitamin C. *Canadian Med. Assoc.* **111**, 31-36.

Anderson, R. and Nilsson, K. (1972). Cyclic-AMP and calcium in relaxation in intestinal smooth muscle. *Nature New Biol.* **238**, 119-120.

Angles d'Auriac, G. and Meyer, P. (1972). Effects of angiotensin II on cyclic 3'5' AMP in rat uterus. *Life Sciences* **11**, Part I, 631-641.

Anitschkow, N. (1933). *In* "Atherosclerosis", p. 291 (Ed. E. V. Cowdry). Macmillan, New York.

Arnaud, C. D., Jr., Tenenhouse, A. M. and Rasmussen, H. (1967). Parathyroid hormone. *Ann Rev. Physiology* **29**.

Assem, E. S. K. and Schild, H. O. (1969). Inhibition by sympathomimetic amines of histamine release induced by antigen in passively sensitised human being. *Nature* **224**, 1028-1029.

Atkins, G. L., Dean, B. M., Griffin, W. J. and Watts, R. W. E. (1964). Quantitiative aspects of ascorbic acid metabolism in man. *J. Biol. Chem.* **239**, 2975-2980.

Austen, K. F. and Lichtenstein, L. M. (1973). "Asthma. Physiology, Pharmacology and Treatment", Academic Press, London and New York.

Avery, E. C., Remko, J. R. and Smalle, R. B. (1968). EPR Dectection of hydrated electron in water. *J. Chem. Phys.* **49**, 951.

B

Bailey, C. W., Bright, J. R. and Jasper, J. J. (1945). A study of the binary system nicotinamide-ascorbic acid. *J. Amer. Chem. Soc.* **67**, 1184–1186.

Baker, E. M. (1967). Vitamin C requirements in stress. *Amer. J. Clin. Nutrition* **20**, 6, 583–593.

Baker, E. M., Bierman, E. L. and Plough, I. C. (1960). Effect of D-glucuronic acid and D-glucuronolactone on ascorbic acid levels in blood and urine of man and dog. *Amer. J. Clin. Nutrition* **8**, 369–373.

Ba r, E. M., Bierman, E. L. and Plough, I. C. (1960). Factors influencing urinary excretion of ketopentoses in normal man. *Metabolism* **9**, 478–483.

Baker, E. M., Hammer, D. C., March, S. C., Tolbert, B. M. and Canham, J. E. (1971). Ascorbate sulfate: A urinary metabolite of ascorbic acid in man. *Science* **173**, 826–827.

Baker, E. M., Hodges, R. E., Hood, J., Sauberlich, H. E. and March, S. C. (1969). *Amer. J. Clin. Nutrition* **22**, 549–558.

Baker, E. M., Levandoski, N. G. and Sauberlich, H. E. (1963). Respiratory catabolism in man of the degradative intermediates of L-ascorbic-1-C^{14} acid. *Proc. Soc. Exptl. Biol. Med.* **113**, 2, 379–383.

Baker, E. M., Levandoski, N. G. and Sauberlich, H. E. (1964). Respiratory catabolism in man of the degradative intermediates of L-ascorbic-1-C^{14} acid. *Nutr. Abstracts & Reviews* **34**, 195.

Baker, E. M., Saari, J. C. and Tolbert, B. M. (1966). Ascorbic acid metabolism in man. *Amer. J. Clin. Nutrition* **19**, 371–378.

Baker, E. M., Sauberlich, H. E., Wolfskill, S. J., Wallace, W. T. and Dean, E. E. (1962). Tracer studies of vitamin C utilisation in man: Metabolism of D-glucuronolactone-6-C^{14}, D-glucuronic-6-C^{14} acid and L-ascorbic acid-1-C^{14} acid. *Proc. Soc. Exptl. Biol. Med.* **109**, 737–741.

Baker, E. M., Sauberlich, H. E., Amos, W. H. and Tillotson, S. A. (1966). Use of carbon-14 labeled vitamins in human nutrition studies: Pyridoxine and L-ascorbic acid. *Amer. J. Clin. Nutrition* **18**, 302–303.

Ball, E. G. (1937). Studies on oxidation-reduction. XXIII. Ascorbic acid. *J. Biol. Chem.* **118**, 219–239.

Banks, H. S. (1968). Controlled trials in the early antibiotic treatment of colds. *The Medical Officer* **119**, 7–10.

Barnes, F. E. (1961). Vitamin C supplements and the incidence of colds in High School basketball players. *N. Carolina Med. J.* **22**, 22–26.

Barnes, M. J. and Kodicek, E. (1972). Biological hydroxylations and ascorbic acid with special regard to collagen metabolism. *Vitamins and Hormones* **30**, (Eds. R. S. Harris, P. L. Munson, J. Glover and E. Dkzfalusy).

Barr, N. F. and King, C. G. (1956). The γ-ray induced oxidation of ascorbic acid and ferrous ion. *J. Amer. Chem. Soc.* **78**, 303–5.

Bartelheimer, H. (1939). Das Vitamin C in der Diabetesbehandlung. *Med. Welt.* **13**, 117–120.

Baur, Von, H. and Staub, H. (1954). Herotitistherapie mit Ascorbinsaüreinfusionen. Vergleich mit anderen Therapien. Schweiz. *Med. Wschr.* **84**, 595–597.

Beauvillain, A. and Sarradin, J. (1948). L'ascorbate d'adrénaline. Etude spectrographique des produits d'oxydation à l'air. *Bull. Ste. Chim. Biol.* **30**, 472–478.

Beavo, J. A., Hardman, J. G. and Sutherland, E. W. (1970). Hydrolysis of cyclic guanosine and adenosine 3′,5′-monophosphates by rat and bovine tissues. *J. Biol. Chem.* **245**, 5649–5655.

Becker, R. R., Burch, H. B., Solomon, L. L., Venkitasubramanian, T. A. and King, C. G. (1953). Ascorbic acid deficiency and cholesterol synthesis. *J. Amer. Chem. Soc.* **75**, 2020.

Banade, L., Howard, T. and Burk, D. (1969). Synergistic killing of Ehrlich ascites carcinoma cells by ascorbate and 3-amino-1,2,4-triazole. *Oncology* **23**, 33–43.

Berthet, J. (1960). Action du glucagon sur le métabolisme des lipides dans le tissue renatique. Proc. 4th Int. Cong. Biochem. **17**, section 9, 107.

Bessey, O. A. and King, C. G. (1933). The distribution of vitamin C in plant and animal tissues, and its determination. *J. Biol. Chem.* **103**, 687–698.

Bezssonoff, M. N. and Woloszyn, M. (1938). Sur l'existence d'une forme oxydee, intermediaire entre la vitamin C et l'acide dehydroascorbique. *Bull. Soc. Chim. Biol.* **20**, 93–122.

Bietti, G. (1935). La Vitamina C (acido ascorbico) nei liquidi e tessuti oculari; suoi rapporti colla biologia del cristallino. *Bull. Occulist*, **14**, 3–33.

Birch, T. W. and Harris, L. J. (1933). The titration curve and dissociation constants of vitamin C. *Biochem. J.* **27**, 595–597.

Bloch, M. (Jan. 1973). Magnesium depletion: Possible significance in ischaemic heart disease. *Brit. J. Hosp. Med.* 91–98.

Blois, M. S. (1958). Antioxidant determinations by the use of a stable free radical. *Nature* (April), **181**, No. 4617, 1199–1200.

Blumberg, W. E., Goldstein, M., Lauber, E. and Peisach, J. (1965). Magnetic resonance studies on the mechanism of the enzymatic β-hydroxylation of 3:4-dihydroxyphenylethylanine. *Biochim. Biophys. Acta* **99**, 187–190.

Borg, D. C. (1965). Transient free radical forms of hormones: EPR spectra from catecholamines and adrenochrome. *Proc. N.A.S.* **53**, 633–639.

Borg, D. (1965). Transient free radical forms of hormones: EPR spectra from iodothyronines, indoles, estrogens, and insulin. *Proc. Natn. Acad. Sci.* **53**, 829–836.

Borsook, H., Davenport, H. W., Jeffreys, C. E. P. and Warner, R. C. (1937). The oxidation of ascorbic acid and its reduction in vitro and in vivo. *J. Biol. Chem.* **117**, 237–279.

Brana, H. and Chytil, F. (1966). Splitting of cyclic 3′-5′-nucleotide phosphodiesterase in a cell-free system of Escherichia Coli. *Folia Microbiologica* **11**, 43-48.

Bourne, H. R., Tomkins, G. M. and Dion, S. (1973). Regulation of phospho-diesterase synthesis: Requirement for cyclic adenosine monophosphate-dependent protein kinase. *Science* **181**, 952–953.

Briggs, M. H. (1962). Malnutrition and mental disease. *Brit. Med. J.* **I**, 1078.

Briggs, M. H. (1973). Vitamin C and infertility. *Lancet* (Sept.), 677–678.

Briggs, M. H. (1973). Vitamin C and colds. *Lancet* (May), 998.

Briggs, M. H., Garcia-Webb, P. and Davies, P. (1973). Urinary oxalate and vitamin C supplements. *Lancet* (July), **II**, 201.

Briggs, M. H., Garcia-Webb, P. and Johnson, J. (1973). Dangers of excess vitamin C. *Medical Journal of Australia* **2**, 48–49.

Broadus, A. E., Kaminsky, N. I., Northcutt, R. C., Hardman, J. G., Sutherland, E. W. and Liddle, G. W. (1970). Effects of glucagon on adenosine $3',5'$-monophosphate and guanosine $3',5'$-monophosphate in human plasma and urine. *J. Clin. Invest.* **49**, 2237–2245.

Brodie, B. B. and Costa, E. (1962). Some current views on brain monoamines. *Psychopharmacol. Serv. Center Bull.* **2**, 1–25.

Bublitz, C., Grollman, A. P. and Lehninger, A. L. (1957). Enzymatic conversion of D-glucuronate to L-ascorbate in animal tissues. *Fed. Proc.* **16**, 382.

Brooker, G., Thomas, L. J. and Appleman, M. M. (1968). The assay of adenosine $3',5'$-cyclic monophosphate and guanosine $3',5'$-cyclic monophosphate in biological materials by enzymatic radioisotopic displacement. *Biochemistry* **7**, 4177.

Buck, M. G. and Zadunaisky, J. A. (1975). Stimulation of ion transport by ascorbic acid through inhibition of $3':5'$-cyclic-AMP phosphodiesterase in the corneal epithelium and other tissues. *Biochim. Biophys. Acta* **389**, 251–260.

Burlamacchi, L. and Tiezzi, E. (1971). Electron paramagnetic resonance of free radicals in hydrazine involving processes. "Magnetic Resonance in Biological Research", pp. 199–201. (Ed. C. Franconi). Gordon and Breach, Pub.

Burns, J. J. (1957). Biosynthesis of L-gulonic acid in rats and guinea pigs. *J. Amer. Chem. Soc.* **74**, 1257.

Burns, J. J. (1967). Ascorbic acid, Chapter 7. "Metabolic Pathways", Vol. I, 3rd Edn (Ed. D. H. Greenberg). Academic Press, London and New York.

Burns, J. J., Burch, H. B. and King, C. G. (1951). The metabolism of $1\text{-}C^{14}$-L-ascorbic acid in guinea pigs. *J. Biol. Chem.* **191**, 501–514.

Burns, J. J., Dayton, P. G. and Eisenberg, F. (1957). Metabolism of L-gulono-lactone in rats via pentose formation. *Biochim. Biophys. Acta* **25**, 647–648.

Burns, J. J. and Evans, C. (1956). The synthesis of L-ascorbic acid in the rat from D-glucuronolactone and L-gulonolactone. *J. Biol. Chem.* **223**, 897–905.

Burns, J. J., Kanger, J. and Dayton, P. G. (1958). Metabolism of L-ascorbic acid in rat kidney. *J. Biol. Chem.* **232**, 107–115.

Burns, J. J. and Mosbach, E. H. (1956). Further observations on the biosynthesis of L-ascorbic acid from D-glucose in the rat. *J. Biol. Chem.* **227**, 107–111.

Burns, J. J., Peyser, P. and Moltz, A. (1956). Missing step in guinea pigs required for the biosynthesis of L-ascorbic acid. *Science* **124**, 1148–1149.

Burk, R. R. (1968). Reduced adenyl cyclase activity in a polyoma virus transformed cell line. *Nature* **219**, 1272–1275.

Businco, L. (1949). Azioni Antistaminiche Nei Tessuti. *Bolletino Societa Italiana Di Biologia Sperimentale* **25**, 274–276.

Busing, M. K. (1942). Der Wirkungsmechanismus der 1-Ascorbinsäure in Stoffwechsel und Messenchym. *Klinische Wochenschrift* **21**, 97‑100.

C

Caels, F. (1953). Contribution a l'étude de l'effet de hautes doses de vitamine C dans les infections oto-rhino-laryngologiques. *Acta Oto-Rhino-Laryngologica Belgica* **7**, 395‑410.

Cameron, E. and Pauling, L. (1973). Ascorbic acid and the glycosaminoglycans. *Oncology* **27**, 181‑192.

Chan, P. C., Becker, R. R. and King C. G. (1958). Metabolic products of L-ascorbic acid. *J. Biol. Chem.* **281**, 231‑240.

Charleston, S. S. and Clegg, K. M. (1972). Ascorbic acid and the common cold. *Lancet* **1**, 1401‑1402.

Chatterjee, I. B. (1973). Evolution and the biosynthesis of ascorbic acid. *Science* (Dec.), 1271‑1272.

Chatterjee, I. B. (1973). Vitamin C synthesis in animals: Evolutionary trend. *Science and Culture* **39**, 210‑212.

Chatterjee, I. B. (1970). Biosynthesis of L-ascorbate in animals. *Methods Enzymol.* **18**, Pt.A. 28‑34.

Chatterjee, I. B., Chatterjee, G. C., Ghosh, N. C., Ghosh, J. J. and Guha, B. C. (1960). Biological synthesis of L-ascorbic acid in animal tissues: Conversion of L-gulonolactone and L-ascorbic acid. *Biochem. J.* **74**, 193‑202.

Chatterjee, I. B., Ghosh, N. C., Ghosh, J. J. and Guha, B. C. (1957). Effect of cyanide on biosynthesis of ascorbic acid *in vitro*. *Science* **126**, 608‑609.

Chatterjee, I. B., Ghosh, J. J., Ghosh, N. C. and Guha, B. C. (1958). Effect of cyanide on the biosynthesis of ascorbic acid by an enzyme preparation from goat-liver tissue. *Biochem. J.* **70**, 509‑515.

Chatterjee, I. B., Kar, N. C., Ghosh, N. C. and Guha, B. C. (1961). Biosynthesis of L-ascorbic acid: Missing steps in animals incapable of synthesising the vitamin. *Nature* **192**, 163‑164.

Chatterjee, G. C., Majunder, P. K., Banergee, S. K., Ray, R. K., Ray, B. and Rudrapal, D. (1975). Relationship of protein and mineral intake to ascorbic acid metabolism, including considerations of some directly related hormones. Second International Conference on Vitamin C held in New York on 9‑12 Oct., 1974. *Ann. N.Y. Acad. Sci.* (1975, in press).

Chatterjee, I. B., Majunder, A. K., Nandi, B. K. and Subramanian, N. (1974/5). The synthesis and some major functions of vitamin C in animals. Abstracts of the Second Conference on Vitamin C held in New York on 9‑12 Oct. 1974. *Ann. N.Y. Acad. Sci.* (1975, in press).

Chaudhuri, C. R. and Chatterjee, I. B. (1969). L-ascorbic acid synthesis in birds: Phylogenetic trend. *Science* **164**, 435‑436.

Cheraskin, E., Ringsdorf, W. M., Michael, D. W. and Hicks, B. S. (1973). Daily vitamin C consumption and reported respiratory findings. *Internat. J. Vit. Nutr. Res.* **43**, 42–55.

Cheung, W. Y. (1970). Cyclic 3′,5′-nucleotide phosphodiesterase: demonstration of an activator. *Biochem. Biophys. Res. Commun.* **38**, 533–538.

Cheung, W. Y. and Patrick, S. (1970). A protein activator of cyclic 3′,5′-nucleotide phosphodiesterase. *Fed. Proceed.* **29**, 602.

Cheung, W. Y. and Salganicoff, L. (1966). Subcellular localization of a cyclic 3′,5′-nucleotide phosphodiesterase in rat brain. *Fed. Proceedings* **25**, 714.

Christine, L., Thomson, G., Iggo, B., Brownie, A. C. and Stewart, C. P. (1956). The reduction of dehydroascorbic acid by human erythrocytes. *Clinica Chim. Acta* **1**, 557–569.

Comfort, A., Youhotsky-Gore, I. and Pathmanathan, K. (1971). Effect of ethoxyquin on the longevity of C3H mice. *Nature* **229**, 254–255.

Conney, A. H., Bray, G. A., Evans, C. and Burns, J. J. (1961). Metabolic interactions between L-ascorbic acid and drugs. *Ann. N.Y. Acad. Sci.* **92**, 115–127.

Consolazio, C. F., Johnson, R. E. and Pecora, L. J. (1960). *In* "Physiological Measurements of Metabolic Functions", p. 437. McGraw-Hill, New York.

Conney, A. H. and Burns, J. J. (1961). Metabolism of uridine diphosphate glucuronic acid by liver and kidney. *Biochim. Biophys. Acta* **54**, 369–372.

Cottingham, E. and Mills, C. A. (1943). Influence of environmental temperature and vitamin-deficiency upon phagocytic functions. *J. Immunology* **47**, 493–502.

Coulehan, J. L., Reiseinger, K. S., Rogers, K. D. and Bradley, D. W. (1974). Vitamin C prophylaxis in a boarding school. *New England J. Med.* **290**, 6–10.

Cowan, D. W., Diehl, H. S. and Baker, A. B. (1942). Vitamins for the prevention of colds. Maximum dose of 500 mg vitamin C. *J. Amer. Med. Assoc.* **120**, 1268–1271.

Cox, E. G., Hirst, E. L. and Reynolds, R. J. W. (1932). Hexuronic acid as the antiscorbutic factor. *Nature* (Dec.), **130**, 3293, 888.

Crozier, D. H., Dickinson, J. R. and Swoboda, B. E. P. (1974). Multiple adenosine 3′:5′-cyclicmonophosphate-binding proteins of the adrenal cortex. *Biochem. Soc. Trans.* **2**, 415–416.

Curtin, C. and King, C. G. (1955). The metabolism of ascorbic acid-1-C[14] and oxalic acid-C[14] in the rat. *J. Biol. Chem.* **216**, 539–548.

D

Dahn, H., Loewe, L. and Bunton, C. A. (1960). Über die Oxydation von Ascorbinsäure durch salpetrige Säure der Einfluss von Azid-ionen. *Helv. Chim. Acta* **XLIII**, No. 40–41, 317–333.

Dahn, H., Loewe, L., Luscher, E. and Menasse, R. (1960). Über die Oxydation von Ascorbinsäure durch salpetrige Säure. I. Stochiometrie und kinetische Messtechnik. *Helvetia Chimica Acta* **XLIII**, 1, No. 37, 287–293.

Dainow, I. (1943). Traitement du zona par la vitamine C. *Dermatologia* **68**, 197-201.

Dalton, W. L. (1962). Massive doses of vitamin C in the treatment of viral diseases. *J. Indiana State Medical Asscn.* **55**, 8, 1151-1154.

Dawson, W. and West, G. B. (1965). The influence of ascorbic acid on histamine metabolism in guinea pigs. *Brit. J. Pharmacol.* **24**, 725-734.

Dawson, W., Hemsworth, B. A. and Stockham, M. A. (1967). Actions of sodium ascorbate on smooth muscle. *Br. J. Pharmac. Chemotherapeutics* **31**, 269-275.

Dayton, P. G., Eisenberg, F. and Burns, J. J. (1959). Metabolism of C^{14} labeled ascorbic, dehydroascorbic and diketogulonic acids in guinea pigs. *Arch. Biochem. Biophys.* **81**, 111-118.

De Fabro, S. P. (1968). Activite de la gulone-lactone-oxydase chez l'embryon de Cobaye. *Comptes Rendu des Seances de la Societe de Biologie et de ses Filiales* **162**, 284-285.

Degkwitz, von E., Schneider, W. and Staudinger, H. J. (1964/5). Biochemie der Ascorbinsäure. *In* "Ascorbinsäure", 11th Symposium in Mainz 2-3 April 1964, in Wissenschaftliche Veröffentlichungen der deutschen Gesellschaft für Ernährung, Vol. 14 (1964). Dr. Dietrich Steinkopf Verlag, Darmstadt, pp. 17-60.

Denisov, B. M. (1964). Effect of the oxidation products of catecholamines on the ATP-ase activity of myosine. *UKR. Biochem. J.* **36**, 711-717.

Deucher, W. G. (1940). Beobachtungen über den Vitamin-C-Haushalt bei Tumorkranken. *Strahlentherapie* **67**, 143-151.

Dick, J. F. and Daniel, C. W. (1973). The hypoglycemic effect of ascorbic acid in a juvenile-onset diabetic. International Research Communication System, 10-19-1.

Dische, Z. and Zil, H. (1951). Studies on the oxidation of cysteine to cystine in lens proteins during cataract formation. *Am. J. Ophthalmology* **38**, 104-113.

Duke, P. S. (1968). Relation of melanoma homogenate and ascorbate solution electron paramagnetic resonance doublets. *Experimental and Molecular Pathology* **8**, 112-122.

Dykes, M. H. M. and Meier, P. (1975). Ascorbic acid and the common cold. *J. Amer. Med. Assoc.* **231**, 1073-1079.

E

Earp, H. S., Watson, B. S. and Ney, R. L. (1969). Adenosine-3′,5′-monophosphate (cyclic AMP) as the mediator of ACTH induced depletion of ascorbic acid in the adrenal cortex. *Clinical Research* **17**, 22.

Earp, H. S., Watson, B. S. and Ney, R. L. (1970). Adenosine 3′,5′-monophosphate as the mediator of ACTH-induced ascorbic acid depletion in the rat adrenal. *Endocrinology* **87**, 118-123.

Edgar, J. A. (1970). Dehydroascorbic acid and cell division. *Nature* **227**, 24-26.

Edlbacher, S. and Von Segesser, A. (1937). Der Abbau des Histidins und anderer Imidazole durch Ascorbinsäure. *Biochemische Zeitschrift* 290, 37, 377.

Einhauser, M. (1939). Giftwirkung der Schlafmittel und Nebennierenrinde. *Klin. Wochenschrift* 18, 423-427.

Eisenberg, F. Jr., Dayton, P. G. and Burns, J. J. (1959). Studies on the glucuronic acid pathway of glucose metabolism. *J. Biol. Chem.* 234, 250-253.

Elliott, C. G. and Smith, M. D. (1966). Ascorbic acid metabolism and glycolysis in the polymorphonuclear leucocyte of the guinea pig. *J. Cellular Physiology* 67, 1, 169-175.

Emmer, M., Crombrugghe, B., Pastan, I. and Perlman, R. (1970). Cyclic AMP receptor protein of E. coli: its role in the synthesis of inducible enzymes. *Proc. Nat. Acad. Sci.* 66, 480-487.

Eufinger, H. and Gaehtgens, G. (1936). Über die Einwirkung des Vitamin C auf das pathologisch veränderte weisse Blutbild. *Klinische Wochenschrift* 15, 150-151.

Euler, von, H. V. and Malmberg, M. (1936). Neue Versuche über Ascorbinsaüre (C-vitamin) in tierischen Augenlinsen. *Arch. Augenheilkund.* 109, 225-234.

Euler, von, H. V. and Klussman, E. (1934). Hochreduzierende Zwischenprodukte (Reduktone) bei der alkalischen Umwandlung einfacher Zuckerarten. *Ark. kem. Mineral. Geol.* 47, 11B, 1-6.

Evans, C., Conney, A. H., Trousof, N. and Burns, J. J. (1960). Metabolism of D-galactose to D-glucuronic acid, L-gulonic acid and L-ascorbic acid in normal and barbital-treated rats. *Biochim. Biophys. Acta* 41, 9-14.

Evans, H. J. and McAuliffe, C. (1956). Identification of NO, N_2O, and N_2 as products of the non-enzymatic reduction of nitrite by ascorbate or reduced diphosphopyridine nucleotide. Symposium on Inorganic Nitrogen Metabolism (Ed. W. D. McElroy and B. Glass). Johns Hopkins Press, Baltimore.

Everling, F. B., Weis, W. and Staudinger, H. (1969). Bestimmung des Standardredoxypotentials (pH 7.0) von L-(+)-Ascorbat/Semidehydro-L(+)-Ascorbinsäure durch nichtenzymatische reaktion von L(+)-Ascorbat/Semidehydro-L(+)-Ascorbinsäure mit Cytochrom $b_5(Fe^2)$/Cytochrom $b_5(Fe^3)$. *Hoppe-Seyler's Z. Physiol. Chem.* 350, 886-888.

F

Fiddick, R. and Heath, H. (1967). The separation of bound ascorbic acid from rat adrenals by gel filtration. *Biochim. Biophys. Acta* 136, 206-213.

Foerster, G. V., Weis, W. and Staudinger, H. (1965). Messung der Elektronenspinresonanz an Semidehydroascorbinsäure. *Ann. Chem.* 690, 166-169.

Fontana, V. J., Salanitro, A. S., Wolfe, H. I. and Moreno, F. (1965). Bacterial vaccine and infectious asthma. *J. Amer. Med. Assoc.* 193, 895-900.

Frank, M. and de Vries, A. (1966). Prevention of urolithiasis. *Arch. Environ. Health* 13, 625-630.

Frankland, A. W. and Howard-Hughes, W. (1955). Atogenous vaccines bacterial in treatment of asthma. *Brit. Med. J.* (Oct.), 941-944.

Franz, W. L., Sands, G. W. and Heyl, H. L. (1956). Blood ascorbic acid level in bioflavonoid and ascorbic acid therapy of common cold. *J. Amer. Assoc.* **162**, 1224–1226.

Friedman, G., Sherry, S. and Ralli, E. P. (1940). The mechanism of the excretion of vitamin C by the human kidney at low and normal plasma levels of ascorbic acid. *J. Clinical Invest.* **19**, 685–689.

Friedman, R. M. and Pastan, I. (1969). Interferon and cyclic $3',5'$-adenosine monophosphate: potentiation of antiviral activity. *Biochem. biophys. Res. Commun.* **36**, 735–740.

G

Gaehtgens, G. (1938). Das Vitamin-C Defizit bei gynakologischem Karzinom. *Zbl. Gynak* **34**, 1874–1881.

General Practitioner Trials (1968). Ineffectiveness of Vitamin C in treating coryza. *Practitioner* **200**, 442–445.

Gericke, D. and Chandra, P. (1969). Inhibition of tumor growth by nucleoside cyclic $3',5'$-monophosphates. *Hoppe-Seyler's Z. Physiol. Chem.* **350**, 1469–1471.

Gero, E. and Le Gallic, P. (1952). Le Mecanisme de l'oxydation de l'acide L-ascorbique. *Compt. Rendu* **234**, 145–147.

Gershoff, S. N. (1964). The formation of urinary stones. *Metabolism* **13**, 875–887.

Ginter, E., Kajaba, I. and Nizner, O. (1970). The effect of ascorbic acid on cholesterolemia in healthy subjects with seasonal deficit of vitamin C. *Nutr. Metabol.* **12**, 76–86.

Glazebrook, A. J. and Thompson, S. (1942). The administration of vitamin C in a large institution and its effect on general health and resistance to infection. *J. Hygiene* **42**(1), 1–19.

Goldberg, N. D., Haddox, M. K., Dunham, E., Lopez, C. and Hadden, J. W. (1973). Evidence for opposing influences of cyclic GMP and cyclic AMP in the regulation of cell proliferation and other biological processes. Cold Spring Harbor Meeting on Proliferation in Animal Cells (1973), p. 40.

Goldsmith, G. A. (1961). Human requirements for vitamin C and its use in clinical medicine. *Ann. N.Y. Acad. Sci.* **92**, 230–245.

Goldsmith, G. A. (1971). Common cold: Prevention and treatment with ascorbic acid not effective. *J. Amer. Med. Assoc.* **216**, 337.

Goldstein, M. L. (1971). High dose ascorbic acid therapy. *J. Amer. Med. Assoc.* **216**, 332–333.

Gontzea, J., Dumitrache, S., Rujinski, A. and Cocora, D. (1963). Der Bedarf an Vitamin C bei Bleiarbeitern. *Int. Z. angew. Physiol. Cinschl. Arbeitsphysiol.* **20**, 20–23.

Gordonoff, T. (1960). Darf man wasserlösliche Vitamine überdosieren? *Schweizerische Med. Wochenschrift* **90**, 726–729.

Goren, E., Erlichman, J., Rosen, O. M. and Rosen, S. M. (1970). A possible role for cyclic nucleotide phosphodiesterase in the regulation of the intracellular concentration of cyclic $3',5'$-AMP. *Fed. Proceed.* **29**, 602 Abs, 1995.

Goth, A. and Littman, I. (1948). Ascorbic acid content in human cancer tissue. *Cancer research* (Aug.), **8**, 349–351.

Gould, B. S. (1970). Possible folate ascorbate interaction in collagen formation. *In* "Chemistry and Molecular Biology of the Intercellular Matric", vol. 1, pp. 431–437 (Ed. E. A. Balazs). Academic Press, New York.

Grimble, R. F. and Hughes, R. E. (1967). A "dehydroascorbic acid reductase" factor in guinea pig tissues. *Experientia* **23**, 362.

Gupta, S. D., Gupta, C. S., Chaudhuri, C. R. and Chatterjee, I. B. (1970). Enzymatic synthesis of L-ascorbic acid from synthetic and biological D-glucurono-1,4-lactone conjugates. *Analyt. Biochem.* **38**, 46–55.

Gupta, S. D., Chaudhuri, C. R. and Chatterjee, I. B. (1972). Incapability of L-ascorbic acid synthesis by insects. *Arch. Biochem. Biophys.* **152**, 889–890.

Guttman, D. E. and Brooke, D. (1963). Solution phase interaction of nicotinamide with ascorbic acid. *J. Pharmaceutical Sciences* **52**, 941–945.

H

Hara, T. and Minakami, S. (1969). According to Iyanagi, T. and Yamazaki, I. *Biochim. Biophys. Acta* **172**, 370–381. Proc. Symp. on Enzyme Chem. Kanazawa (1968) p. 21 (Japanese).

Harris, L. J. (1935). "Vitamins in Theory and in Practice". Cambridge University Press.

Hassan, M. U. and Lehninger, A. L. (1956). Enzymatic formation of ascorbic acid in rat liver extracts. *J. Biol. Chem.* **223**, 123–138.

Hausen, H. Z. (1975). Oncogenic herpes viruses. *Biochim. Biophys. Acta* **417**, 25–53.

Haworth, W. N. and Hirst, E. L. (1933a). Synthesis of ascorbic acid. *Chemistry and Industry* (4 Aug.), 645–646.

Haworth, W. N. and Hirst, E. L. (1933b). Synthesis of ascorbic acid. *J. Soc. Chem. Industry* **52**, 645–646.

Heacock, R. A. and Powell, W. S. (1973). Adenochrome and related compounds. *Progress in Medical Chemistry* **9**, 275–339.

Heath, H., Beck, T. C. and Rutter, A. C. (1966). Biochemical changes in aphaskia. *Vision Res.* **1**, 274–286.

Heath, H. (1962). The distribution and possible functions of ascorbic acid in the eye. *Exp. Eye Res.* **1**, 362–367.

Heinild, A. S. and Schiodt, E. (1936). Remission under Forlobet af Leukaemi. *Ugeskrift for Laeger* **98**, 1135–1136.

Hellman, L. and Burns, J. J. (1958). Metabolism of L-ascorbic acid-1-C^{14} in man. *J. Biol. Chem.* **230**, 923-930.

Hendrickx, H. and De Moor, H. (1964). Effect of light from fluorescent lamps on the light flavour and ascorbic acid content of milk. *Nutrition Abs.*, **34**, 90.

Herbert, V. and Jacob, E. (1974). Destruction of vitamin B_{12} by ascorbic acid. *J. Amer. Med. Assoc.* **230**, 2, 241–242.

Herbert, R. W., Hirst, E. L., Percival, E. G. V., Reynolds, R. J. W. and Smith, F. (1933). The constitution of ascorbic acid. *J. Chem. Soc.* 1270–1290.

Hermann-Erlee, M. P. N., Hekkelman, J. W., Heersche, Y. N. M. and Nijweide, P. J. (1975). The role of Ca^{++} and cyclic AMP in the action of parathyroid hormone on embryonic bone in vitro. *J. Endocrinol.* **64** (3), 69p.

Hewitt, E. J. and Dicks, G. J. (1961). Spectrophotometric measurements on ascorbic acid and their use for the estimation of ascorbic acid and dehydro-ascorbic acid in plant tissues. *Biochem. J.* **78**, 384–391.

Hoffer, A. (1973). Vitamin C and infertility. *Lancet* (17 Nov.), p. 1146.

Hoffer, A. and Osmond, H. (1963). Scurvy and schizophrenia. Diseases of the Nervous System, **XXIV**, 273–285.

Hoffer, A. and Osmond, H. (1967). "The Hallucinogens", Academic Press, New York and London.

Holden, M. and Resnick, R. (1936). The *in vitro* action of synthetic crystalline vitamin C (ascorbic acid) on herpes virus. *J. Immunol.* **31**, 455–462.

Holden, M. and Molloy, E. (1937). Further experiments on the inactivation of herpes virus by vitamin C (L-ascorbic acid). *J. Immunol.* **33**, 251–257.

Hollman, S. and Touster, O. (1957). The L-xylulose-xylitol enzyme and other polyol dehydrogenases of guinea pig liver mitochondria. *J. Biol. Chem.* **225**, 87–102.

Holtz, P. (1937). Über den Mechanismus des Histidinabbaus durch Ascorbin-säure und Thioglykolsäure. *Z. Physiol. Chem.* **250**, 87.

Holtz, P. and Westermann, E. (1956). Über die Histindecarboxylase der Nerven. *Naturwissenschaften* **43**, 37.

Hopkins, F. G. (1937). The influence of lactoflavin as a promoter of the photocatalytic oxidation of ascorbic acid. *J. Soc. Chem. Industry* **56**, 934.

Hornick, R. B. (1972). Does ascorbic acid have value in combating the common cold? *Med. Counterpoint* **4**, 50–56.

Hornig, D., Weber, F. and Wiss, O. (1974). Influence of erythorbic acid on the vitamin C status in guinea pigs. *Experientia* **30**, 173–174.

Horowitz, H. H. and King, C. G. (1953). The conversion of glucose-6-C^{14} to ascorbic acid by the albino rat. *J. Biol. Chem.* **200**, 125–128.

Horowitz, H. H., Doerschuk, A. P. and King, C. G. (1952). The origin of L-ascorbic acid in the albino rat. *J. Biol. Chem.* **199**, 193–198.

Hughes, R. E. and Maton, S. C. (1968). The passage of vitamin C across the erythrocyte membrane. *Brit. J. Haematol.* **14**, 247–253.

Hume, R. and Weyers, E. (1973). Changes in leucocyte ascorbic acid during the common cold. *Scot. Med. J.* **18**, 3–7.

Hruba, F. and Masek, J. (1962). Einige Aspekte der Wirkung hoher Dosen von L-Ascorbinsäure auf den gesunden Menschen. *Die Nahrung* **6**, 507–517.

Hume, R., Weyers, W., Rowan, T., Reid, D. S. and Hillis, W. S. (1972). Leucocyte ascorbic acid levels after acute myocardial infarction. *Brit. Heart Journal* **34**, 238–243.

Hutchins, H. H., Cravioto, P. J. and Macek, T. J. (1956). A comparison of the stability of cyanocobalamin and its analogs in ascorbate solution. *J. Amer. Pharm. Assoc.* **45**, 806–808.

I

Illiano, G., Tell, G. P., Siegel, M. I. and Cuatrecases, P. (1973). Guanosine 3':5'-cyclic monophosphate and the action of insulin and acetylcholine. *Proc. Nat. Acad. Sci. USA* **70**, 2443–2447.

Inchiosa, M. A. and Freedberg, A. S. (1961). Inhibition of contractile protein ATPase activity by epinephrine oxidized via adrenochrome. *Fed. Proc.* **20**, 298.

Inchiosa, M. A. and Van Demark, N. L. (1958). Influence of oxidation products of epinephrine upon adenosinetriphosphatase activity of uterine muscle preparations. *Proc. Soc. Exptl. Biol. and Med.* **97**, 595–597.

Ingalls, T. H. (1939). Infantile scurvy. Part II. Studies on the concentration of ascorbic acid in the tissues. *J. Pediat.* **14**, 593–601.

Isherwood, F. A., Chen, Y. T. and Mapson, L. W. (1954). Synthesis of L-ascorbic acid in plants and animals. *Biochem. J.* **56**, 1–15.

Iyanagi, T. and Yamazaki, I. (1969). One-electron-transfer reactions in biochemical systems. III. One-electron reduction of quinones by microsomal flavin enzymes. *Biochim. Biophys. Acta* **172**, 370–381.

J

Jackel, S. S., Mosbach, E. H., Burns, J. J. and King, C. G. (1950). The synthesis of L-ascorbic acid by the albino rat. *J. Biol. Chem.* **186**, 569–577.

Jakowlew, N. (1958). Zur Vitaminnorm. *Ernaehrung Forschung* **3**, 446–447.

Jungeblut, C. W. (1935). Inactivation of poliomyelitis virus *in vitro* by crystalline vitamin C (ascorbic acid). *J. Exptl. Med.* **62**, 517–521.

Jungeblut, C. W. (1937). Further observations on vitamin C therapy in experimental poliomyelitis. *J. Exptl. Med.* **66**, 459–477.

Jungeblut, C. W. (1939). A further contribution to vitamin C therapy in experimental poliomyelitis. *J. Exptl. Med.* **70**, 315–332.

K

Kagawa, Y. and Takiguchi, H. (1962). Enzymatic studies on ascorbic acid catabolism in animals. *J. Biochem.* **51**, 3, 197–203.

Kakiuchi, S. and Rall, T. W. (1968). The influence of chemical agents on the accumulation of adenosine 3',5'-phosphate in slices of rabbit cerebellum. *Mol. Pharmacol.* **4**, 367–378. Studies on adenosine 3',5'-phosphate in rabbit cerebral cortex. *Mol. Pharmacol.* **4**, 379–388.

Kamm, J. J., Dashman, T., Conney, A. H. and Burns, J. J. (1973). Protective effect of ascorbic acid on heptatoxicity. *Proc. Nat. Acad. Sci. USA* **70**, 3, 747–749.

Kanfer, J., Ashwell, G. and Burns, J. J. (1960). Formation of L-lyxonic and L-xylonic acids from L-ascorbic acid in the rat kidney. *J. Biol. Chem.* **235**, 2518–2521.

Karlowski, T. R., Frenkel, L. D., Chalmers, T. C., Lynch, J. M., Shaffer, G. W., Kapikian, A. Z., George, D. A. and Lewis, T. L. (1974). Quoted by Lewin, S. in "Chemistry in Britain" (1974).

Karrer, P., Schwarzenbach, K. and Schopp, G. (1933). Über Vitamin C. *Helvetica Chimica Acta* **16**, 302–305.

Kawada, M., Takiguchi, H., Kagawa, Y., Suzuki, K. and Shimazono, N. (1962). Comparative studies on soluble lactonases. *J. Biochem.* **51**, 405–415.

Kenaway, M. R., El-Nabawy El-Mohandis, M. M., El-Dine Rohayem, H. K. and El-Sheehy, A. W. (1952). Studies on the diuretic action of vitamin C in normal animals and human beings, and its clinical value in pathological retention of water. *Internat. Zeitschrift fur Vitaminforschung* **24**, 40–61.

Keller, R. (1972). Suppression of normal and enhanced tumour growth in rats by agents interfering with intracellular cyclic nucleotides. *Life Sciences* **11**, Part II, 4, 485–491.

Kern, M. I. and Racker, E. (1954). Activation of DPNH oxidase by an oxidation product of ascorbic acid. *Arch. Biochem. Biophys.* **48**, 235–236.

Kersten, H., Kersten, W. and Staudinger, Hj. (1956). Zum Wirkungsmechanismus der Ascorbinsäure. *Biochem. Z.* **328**, 24–34.

Kersten, H., Kersten, W. and Staudinger, Hj. (1958). I. Isolierung einer ascorbinsäuren DPNH Oxydase aus Nebennierenmikrosomen. *Biochim. Biophys. Acta* **27**, 598–607.

King, M. C. and Wilson, A. C. (1975). Our close cousin, the chimpanzee. *New Scientist* (3 July), 16–18.

Kirshner, N. and Goodall, McC. (1957). The formation of adrenaline from noradrenaline. *Biochim. Biophys. Acta* **24**, 658–659.

Kirk, J. E. (1962). Variations with age in the tissue content of vitamins and hormones. *Vitamins and Hormones* **20**, 67–139.

Kirchmair, H. and Kirsch, B. (1957). Behandlung der Hepatitis epidemica im Kindesalter mit hohen Dosen Ascorbinsäure. *Mediz. Monatschr.* **11**, 353–357.

Klenner, F. R. (1948). Virus pneumonia and its treatment with vitamin C. *Southern Medicine and Surgery* **10**, 36–38, 46.

Klenner, F. R. (1949). The treatment of poliomyelitis and other virus diseases with vitamin C. *Southern Medicine and Surgery* **111**, 209–214.

Klenner, R. F. (1951). Massive doses of vitamin C and the virus diseases. *Southern Medicine and Surgery* **113**, 101–107.

Klenner, F. R. (1959). The folly in the continued use of a killed polio virus vaccine. *Tri-State Medical Journal* (Feb.), 1–8.

Klenner, F. R. (1971). Observations on the dose and administration of ascorbic acid when employed beyond the range of a vitamin in human pathology. *J. Applied Nutrition* **23**, 61–68.

Kluge, H., Rasch, R., Brux, B. and Frunder, H. (1967). Bildung und Struktur des Ascorbatradikals. *Biochim. Biophys. Acta* **141**, 260–265.

Knight, C. A. and Stanley, W. M. (1944). The effects of some chemicals on purified influenza virus. *J. Exp. Med.* **79**, 291.

Korner, W. F. and Weber, F. (1972). Zur Toleranz hoher Ascorbinsäurendosen. *Internat. Z. Vit. Ernährungsforschung* **42**, 528–544.

Krall, A. R., Siegel, G. J., Gozansky, D. M. and Wagner, F. L. (1964). Adrenochrome inhibition of oxidative phosphorylation by rat brain mitochondria. *Biochem. Pharmacol.* **13**, 1519-1525.

Krisch, K. and Staudinger, Hj. (1959). Zur Wirkung von Ascorbinsäure und Cyrochom b₅ auf die mikrosomale DPNH-Oxydation. *Biochem. Zeitsch.* **331**, 195-208.

Kubler, W. and Gehler, J. (1970). Zur Kinetic der enteralen Ascorbinsäureresorption. Ein beitrag zur Berechnung nicht proportionaler Resorptionsvorgänge. *Internat. Z. Vit. Forschung* **40**, 442-453.

Kumler, W. D. and Daniels, T. C. (1935). Titration curves and dissociation constants of 1-ascorbic acid (vitamin C) and diethyl dihydroxymaleate. *J. Amer. Chem. Soc.* (Oct.) **57**, 1929-1930.

Künzel, O. (1941). X. Die Oberflächenspannung in Serum und Liquor. *Ergebn. Inn. Med. Kinderheilk* **60**, 565-656.

Kyhos, E. D., Sevringhaus, E. L. and Hagedorn, S. (1945). Large doses of ascorbic acid in treatment of vitamin C deficiencies. *Arch. of Internal Medicine* **75**, 407-412.

L

Lagercrantz, C. (1964). Free radicals in the auto-oxidation of ascorbic acid. *Acta Chem. Scand.* **18**, No. 2, 562.

Lamden, M. P. (1971). Dangers of massive vitamin C intake. *New England J. Med.* **284**, 336-337.

Lamden, M. P. and Chrystowski, G. A. (1954). Urinary oxalate excretion by man following ascorbic acid ingestion. *Proc. Soc. Exptl. Biol. and Med.* **85**, 190.

Laufs, R. and Steinke, H. (1975). Vaccination of non-human primates against malignant lymphoma. *Nature* **253**, 71-72.

Lawendel, J. S. (1956). Enhancement of ultra-violet absorption of L-ascorbic acid in the presence of D-sorbitol. *Nature* **178**, 873-874.

Lawendel, J. S. (1957). Ultra-violet absorption spectra of L-ascorbic acid in aqueous solutions. *Nature* **180**, 434-435.

Lavandoski, N. G., Baker, E. M. and Canham, J. E. (1964). A monodehydro form of ascorbic acid in the autoxidation of ascorbic acid to dehydroascorbic acid. *Biochemistry* **3**, 1465-1469.

Leach, B. E., Cohen, M., Heath, R. G. and Martens, S. (1956). Studies of the role of ceruloplasmin and albumin in adrenaline metabolism. *Amer. Med. Assoc. Arch. Neurol. Psychiat.* **76**, 635-642.

Levin, E. Y. and Kaufman, S. (1961). Studies on the enzyme catalysing the conversion of 3-4 dihydroxyphenylethylamine to norepinephrine. *J. Biol. Chem.* **236**, 7, 2043-2049.

Lewin, S. (1960). "The Solubility Product Principle. An Introduction to its Uses and Limitations." Pitman and Sons, London.

Lewin, S. (1971a). New concepts in hydrophilic and hydrophobic water influences on nucleic acid and protein stabilities and interactions. First Eur. Congress of Biophysics, Baden, III, 471–476.

Lewin, S. (1971b). Water surface energy contribution to adherence of hydrophobic groups in relation to stability of protein conformations. *Nature* (*New Biology*) **231**, 80.

Lewin, S. (1974a). "Displacement of Water and its Control of Biochemical Reactions." Academic Press, London and New York.

Lewin, S. (1974b). Vitamin C and the common cold. *Chemistry in Britain* **10**, 25–27.

Lewin, S. (1974c). The use of megaquantities of ascorbic acid or ascorbate for therapeutic and prophylactic purposes in relation to biochemical individuality. *Biochem. Soc. Trans.* **2**, 154–156.

Lewin, S. (1974d). The ascorbate system and the formation of adenosine 38:5′-cyclic monophosphate. *Biochem. Soc. Trans.* **2**, 400–403.

Lewin, S. (1974e). High intake of vitamin C in relation to adenosine 3′:5′-cyclic monophosphate and guanosine 3′:5′-cyclic monophosphate concentrations and to blood sugar concentrations. *Biochem. Soc. Trans.* **2**, 922–924.

Lewin, S. (1974f). Ascorbate requirement and the depression of mental states. *Biochem. Soc. Trans.* **2**, 1080–1082.

Lewin, S. (1974g). Evaluation of the potential effects of high intake of ascorbic acid. *Comp. Biochem. Physiol.* **47B**, 681–695.

Lewin, S. (1974h). Recent advances in the molecular biology of vitamin C. "Vitamin C. Recent aspects of its physiological and technological importance" (Ed. G. G. Birch and K. J. Parker). Applied Science Publishers, Barking, Essex, 221–251.

Lewin, S. (1975a). Transient water free radicals in oxidation-reduction reactions. *Biochem. Soc. Trans.* **3**, 319–321.

Lewin, S. (1975c). Hydrolytic rupture of ascorbate by 3′,5′-cyclic AMP Biochemical Society, Oxford, December. *Biochem. Soc. Trans.*

Lewin, S. (1975c). Hydrolytic rupture of ascorbate by 3′,5′-cyclic AMP Phosphodiesterese. 560th Meeting of the Biochemical Society, Oxford, December. *Biochem. Soc. Trans.*

Lichtenstein, L. M. and Margolis, S. (1968). Histamine release *in vitro* inhibition by catecholamine and methylxanthine. *Science* **161**, 902–903.

Lijinsky, W. and Greenblatt, M. (1972). Carcinogen dimethylnitrosamine produced in vivo from nitrite and aminopyrine. *Nature New Biology* **236**, 177–178.

Linkswiler, H. (1958). The effect of the ingestion of ascorbic acid and dehydroascorbic acid upon the blood levels of these two components in human subjects. *J. Nutrition* **64**, 43–54.

Lloyd, B. B. and Sinclair, H. M. (1953). Chapter 11. Vitamin C. *In* "Biochemical and Physiological Nutrition", Academic Press, New York and London.

Lobova, N. M. (1953). Effect of ascorbic acid on the level of lipo-proteins in blood of patients with atherosclerosis. "Ateroskleroz I Infarkt Miokarda", Medgiz, Moscow, p. 124. Quoted by Simonson, E. and Keys, A. *In* "Clinical progress", *Circulation*, Nov. 1961. Vol. XXIV, pp. 1239–1246.

Loewus, F. A. (1961). Aspects of ascorbic acid biosynthesis in plants. *Ann. N.Y. Acad. Sci.* **92**, 57-78.

Loewus, F. A., Jang, R. and Seegmiller, C. G. (1956). The conversion of C^{14}-labeled sugars to L-ascorbic acid in ripening strawberries. *J. Biol. Chem.* **222**, 649-664.

Loewus, F. A. and Jang, R. (1957). Further studies on the formation of ascorbic acid in plants. *Biochem. Biophys. Acta* **23**, 205-206.

Loh, H. S. (1973). Mortality from atherosclerosis and vitamin C intake. *Lancet* 21 July, 153.

Loh, H. S. and Wilson, C. W. M. (1971). Relationship between leucocyte and plasma ascorbic acid concentrations. *Brit. Med. J.* **3**, 733-735.

Loh, H. S. and Wilson, C. W. M. (1971). The relationship between leucocyte ascorbic acid and haemoglobin levels at different ages. *Internat. J. Vit. Nutr. Res.* **41**, 259-267.

Loh, H. S. and Wilson, C. W. M. (1973). Vitamin C and thrombotic episodes. *Lancet* (11 Aug.), 317.

Lojkin, W. (1936). Inactivation of tobacco mosaic virus by ascorbic acid. Contribution from Boyce Thompson Institute, 8 (Oct. Dec. 1936) No. 4.

Longenecker, H. E., Musulin, R. R., Tully, R. H. and King, C. G. (1939). An acceleration of vitamin C synthesis and excretion by feeding known organic compounds to rats. *J. Biol. Chem.* **129**, 445-453.

Longenecker, H. E., Fricke, H. H. and King, C. G. (1940). The effect of organic compounds upon vitamin C synthesis in the rat. *J. Biol. Chem.* **135**, 497-510.

Lonsdale, K. (1968). Human stones. *Science* **159**, 1199-1207.

Lowry, O. H., Bessey, O. A., Brock, M. J. and Lopez, J. A. (1946). The interrelationship of dietary, serum, white blood cell, and total body ascorbic acid. *J. Biol. Chem.* **166**, 111-119.

Lowry, O. H., Bessey, O. A. and Burch, H. B. (1952). Effects of prolonged high dosage with ascorbic acid. *Proc. Soc. Exptl. Biol.* **80**, 361-362.

M

Major, P. W. and Kilpatrick, R. (1972). Cyclic AMP and hormone action. *J. Endocrin.* **52**, 593-630.

Malaisse, W. J., Malaisse-Lagae, F. and Mayhew, D. (1967). A possible role for the adenylcyclase system in insulin secretion. *J. Clin. Invest.* **46**, 1724-1734.

Mano, Y., Suzuki, K., Yamada, K. and Shimazono, N. (1961). Enzymic studies on TPN L-hexonate dehydrogenase from rat liver. *J. Biochem.* (*Tokyo*) **49**, 618-634.

Mapson, L. W. (1967). Biochemical Systems, pp. 386-398. *In* "The Vitamins", 2nd Edn. (Ed. W. H. Sebrell and R. S. Harris).

Marin, J. V. (1941). Tratamiento experimental de la intoxicacion mercurial aguda en el cobayo por el acido ascorbico. *Revista de le Sociedad Argentina de Biologia* (*Buenos Aires*) **17**, 581-586.

Marchmont-Robinson, S. W. (1941). Effect of vitamin C on workers exposed to lead dust. *J. of Lab. and Clin. Med.* **114**, 1178-1181.

Markwell, N. W. (1947). Vitamin C in the prevention of colds. *Med. J. of Australia* (27 Dec.). **10**, 777-778.

Martin, G. R. (1961). Studies on the tissue distribution of ascorbic acid. *Ann. N.Y. Acad. Sci.* **92**, 141-147.

Mašek, J. and Hrubá, F. (1964). Über die Beziehungen zwischen der Saturation des Serums under der Leukocyten mit Vitamin C. *Int. Z. Vitaminforsch.* **34**, 39-44.

Mattock, G. L. (1965). The mechanism of the reduction of adrenochrome by ascorbic acid. *J. Chem. Soc.* 4728-4735.

McDonald, D. F. and Murphy, G. P. (1959). Bacteriostatic and acidifying effects of methionine, hydrolysed casein and ascorbic acid on the urine. *New England J. Med.* **261**, 803-805.

McIlwain, H., Thomas, J. and Bell, J. L. (1956). The composition of isolated cerebral tissues: Ascorbic acid and cozymose. *Biochem. J.* **64**, 332-335.

McCormick, W. J. (1954). Cancer: The preconditioning factor in pathogenesis. *Arch. Pediat.* **71**, 313-322.

McCormick, W. J. (1963). Cancer: A preventable disease, secondary to a nutritional deficiency. *Clin. Physiol.* **5**, 198-204.

Melka, J. (1936). Über den Ascorbinsäuregehalt (Vitamin C) in verschiedenen Teilen des Zentralnervensystems und in peripheren Nerven.

Merchant, D. J. (1950). The effect of serum on the activity of the polymorphonuclear leucocytes of the guinea pig. *J. Infectious Diseases* **86-87**, 275-284.

Milhorat, T. H. (1944). A colour reaction of ascorbic acid with derivatives of pyridine, piperidine, quinoline, and iso-quinoline. *Proc. Soc. Exptl. Biol. and Med.* **55**, 52-55.

Mills, C. A. (1949). Bone marrow nutrition in relation to the phagocytic activity of blood granulocytes. Effect of ascorbic acid on phagocytic activity established quantitatively. *Blood* **4**, 153-159.

Milner, C. (1963). Ascorbic acid in chronic psychiatric patients—A controlled trial. *Brit. J. Psychiat.* **109**, 294-299.

Mirvish, S. S., Wallcave, L., Eagen, M. and Shubik, P. (1972). Ascorbate-nitrite reaction: Possible means of blocking the formation of carcinogenic N-nitroso compounds. *Science* **177**, 65-68.

Moffat, A. C., Patterson, D. A., Currey, A. S. and Owen, P. (1972). Inhibition *in vitro* of cyclic $3',5'$ nucleotide phosphodiesterase activity by drugs. *European J. Toxicol.* (May-June), **5**(3), 160-162.

Monard, D., Janeck, J. and Rickenberg, H. V. (1969). The enzymic degradation of $3',5'$-cyclic AMP in strains of E. coli sensitive and resistant to catabolite repression. *Biochem. Biophys. Res. Commun.* **35**, 584.

Morton, R. A. (1942). "Application of Absorption Spectra to the Study of Vitamins, Hormones and to Enzymes", Chapter VI, "Vitamin C and Vitamin P." 2nd Edn., pp. 128-135. Hilger and Watts, London.

Mukherjee, S. L. (1959). Stability of vitamin B_{12}. Part II. Protection by an iron salt against destruction by aneurine and nicotinamide. *Jnl. of Pharmacy and Pharmacology* **11**, 26-31.

Murata, A. (1975). Proc. of 1st Intersectional Congress of the International Association of Microbiological Societies, Vol. III. (Tokyo, 1-7 Sept. 1974).

Murata, A. and Kitagawa, K. (1973). Mechanism of inactivation of bacteriophage J1 by ascorbic acid. *Agr. Biol. Chem.* **37**, 5, 1145-1151.

Murata, A., Kitagawa, K. and Saruno, R. (1971). Inactivation of bacteriophages by ascorbic acid. *Agr. Biol. Chem.* **35**, 2, 294-296.

Murata, A., Kitagawa, K., Inmaru, H. and Saruno, R. (1972). Inactivation of bacteriophages by thiol reducing agents. *Agr. Biol. Chem.* **36**, 6, 1065-1067.

Murata, A., Kitagawa, K., Inmaru, H. and Saruno, R. (1972). Inactivation of single stranded DNA and RNA phages by ascorbic acids and thiol reducing agents. *Agr. Biol. Chem.* **36**, 13, 2597-2599.

Murata, A. and Kitagawa, K. (1973). Mechanism of inactivation of bacteriophage J1 by ascorbic acid. *Agr. Biol. Chem.* **37**, 5, 1145-1151.

Murphy, F. J. and Zelman, S. (1965). Ascorbic acid as a urinary acidifying agent: I. Comparison with the ketogenic effect of fasting. *Jnl. Urology* **94**, 297-299.

Musulin, R. R., Tully, R. H., Longenecker, H. E. and King, C. G. (1938). An effect of lipid feeding upon vitamin C excretion by the rat. *Science* **88**, 552.

Myasnikov, A. L. (1958). Influence of some factors on development of experimental cholesterol atherosclerosis. *Circulation* **17**, 99-113.

N

Najer, H. and Guepet, R. (1954). Contribution a l'étude du complexe acide l-ascorbique-nicotinamide: "nicoscorbine". *Ann. Pharm. Franc.* **12**, 712-717.

Nason, A., Wosilait, W. D. and Terrell, A. J. (1954). The enzymic oxidation of reduced pyridine nucleotides by an oxidation product of ascorbic acid. *Arch. Biochem. Biophys.* **48**, 233-235.

Nichelmann, M., Glowatzki, R. and Kemper, A. (1966). Nachweis gebundener Ascorbinsäure in Rattengehirnen. *Acta Biol. Med. German.* **16**, 480-484.

Nungester, W. J. and Ames, A. M. (1948). The relationship between ascorbic acid and phagocytic activity. *J. Infectious Diseases* **83**, 50-54.

O

Ohnishi, T., Yamazaki, H., Iyanagi, T., Nakamura, T. and Yamazaki, I. (1969). One-electron-transfer reactions in biochemical systems. II. The reaction of free radicals formed in the enzymic oxidation. *Biochim. Biophys. Acta* **172**, 357-369.

Oler, A., Lannaccone, P. M. and Gordon, G. B. (1973). Suppression of growth of L cells in suspension culture by dibutyryl adenosine $3',5'$-monophosphate. *In Vitro* **9**, 1, 35-38.

Orr, C. W. M. (1966). The inhibition of catalase by ascorbic acid. *Biochem. Biophys. Res. Commun.* **23**, No. 6, 854-860.

Orr, C. W. M. (1967). Studies on ascorbic acid. I. Factors influencing the ascorbate-mediated inhibition of catalase. *Biochemistry* **6**, 2995–2999.

Orr, C. W. M. (1970). The inhibition of catalase (hydrogen-peroxide: hydrogen peroxide oxireductase, EC 1.11.1.6) by ascorbate. *Methods Enzymol.* **18**, Pt.A. 59–62.

P

Park, J. H., Meriwether, B. P. and Park, C. R. (1956). Effects of adrenochrome on oxidative phosphorylation in liver mitochondria. *Amer. Physiological Soc.* **15**, 141.

Park, J. H., Meriwether, B. P., Mudd, S. H. and Lipmann, F. (1956b). Glutathione and ethylenediaminetetraacetate antagonism of uncoupling oxidative phosphorylation. *Biochim. Biophys. Acta* **22**, 403–404.

Patterson, J. W. (1950). The diabetogenic effect of dehydroascorbic and dehydroisoascorbic acids. *J. Biol. Chem.* **183**, 81–88.

Patterson, J. W. (1949). The diabetogenic effect of dehydroascorbic acid. *Endocrinology* **45**, 344.

Patterson, J. W. (1951). Course of diabetes and development of cataracts after injecting dehydroascorbic acid and related substances. *Am. J. Physiology* **165**, 61–65.

Patterson, J. W. and Mastin, D. W. (1951). Some effects of dehydroascorbic acid on the central nervous system. *Am. J. Physiology* **167**, 119–126.

Paul, M. I., Ditzion, B. R. and Janowsky, D. S. (1970). Effective illness and cyclic AMP excretion. *Lancet* i, 88.

Paul, M. I., Cramer, H. and Bunney, W. E. (1971). Urinary adenosine $3',5'$-monophosphate in the switch process from depression to mania. *Science* **171**, 300–303.

Pauling, L. (1970). "Vitamin C and the Common Cold", W. H. Freeman & Co., San-Francisco.

Pecherer, B. (1951). The preparation of dehydro-L-ascorbic acid and its methanol complex. Some reactions of dehydro-L-ascorbic acid. *J. Amer. Chem. Soc.* **73**, 3827–3830.

Pena, A., Del Arbol, J. L., Torres, J. A. G. and Lara, Y. J. M. (1963). Influencia de la vitamina C sobre la excrecion de acido urico. *Revista Clinica Espanola* **89**, 101–104.

Pena, A., Del Arbol, J. L., Torres, G. J. A. and Lara, M. (1964). Effect of vitamin C on excretion of uric acid. *Nutr. Abstracts and Reviews* **34**, 195–196.

Pfleger, R. and Scholl, F. (1937). Diabetes und Vitamin C. *Wiener Arch. Innere Media.* **31**, 219–229.

Piette, L. H., Yamazaki, I. and Mason, S. H. (1961). Identification of substrate free radical intermediates of peroxidase-substrate oxidation by EPR. *In* "Free Radicals in Biological Systems" (Eds. M. S. Blois, H. W. Brown, *et al.*), pp. 195–208. Academic Press, London and New York.

Pillsbury, S., Watkins, D. and Cooperstein, S. J. (1973). Effect of dehydro-ascorbic acid on permeability of pancreatic islet tissue in vitro. *J. Pharmacol. and Exptl. Therapeutics* **185**, 3, 713-718.

Pirie, A. (1946). Ascorbic acid content of cornea. *Biochem. J.* **40**, 96-99.

Picha, E. and Weghaupt, K. (1956). Über die Behandling mit Vitamin A und C in hohen Dosen bei weit fortgeschrittenen Karzinomen des weiblichen Genital-trakies. *Wiener Medizinische Wochenschrift* Nr. 17, 391-392.

Pitts, R. F., Lospeosch, W. D., Schiess, W. A. and Ayer, J. L. (1948). The renal regulation of acid-base balance in man—I. The nature of the mechanism for acidifying the urine. *J. Clin. Invest.* **27**, 48-56.

Plaut, F. and Bulow, M. (1935). Über Unterschiede im C-Vitamingehalt ver-schiedener Teile des Nervensystems, *Z. ges. Neurol. Psychiat.* **153**, 182-192. [Deutsche Forschunganstalt für Psychiatrie (Kaiser Wilhelm-Institut in München).]

Plum, P. and Thomsen, S. (1936). Remission under Forlobet af Akut, Aleukae-misk Leukaemi. *Ugeskrift for Laeger* **98**, 1062-1067.

Polacek, I. and Daniel, E. E. (1971). Effect of α- and β-adrenergic stimulation of the uterine motility and adenosine $3',5'$-monophosphate level. *Canad. J. Physiol. Pharmacol.* **49**, 988-998.

Polis, B. D., Wyeth, J., Goldstein, L. and Graedon, J. (1969). Stable free-radical forms of plasma proteins or simple related structures which induce brain excitatory effects. *Proc. Natnl. Acad. Sci.* **64**, 755-762.

Poser, E. (1972). Large ascorbic acid intake. *New England J. Med.* **287**, 412.

Price, C. E. (1966). Ascorbate stimulation of RNA synthesis. *Nature* **212**, 1481.

Punekar, P. D. (1961). Blood ascorbic acid levels of mental patients in different age groups: Clinical categories and economic status. *Ind. Jour. Med. Res.* **49**, 828-833.

R

Raiha, N. (1958). On the placental transfer of vitamin C. *Acta Phys. Scand.* **45**, Supp. 155, 5-53.

Rall, T. W. and Kakiuchi, S. (1966). The influence of certain neurohormones and drugs on the accumulation of cyclic $3',5'$-AMP in brain tissue. "Molecu-lar Basis of Some Aspects of Mental Activity," **1**, 417-430.

Ralli, E. P. and Sherry, S. (1940). Effect of insulin on plasma level and excretion of vitamin C. *Proc. Soc. Exptl. Biol and Med.* **43**, 669-672.

Ramp, K. W. and Thornton, P. A. (1968). The effect of ascorbic acid on the glytolytic and respiratory metabolism of embryonic chick tibias. *Calc. Tiss, Res.* **2**, 77-82.

Ramsden, E. N. (1970). Cyclic AMP in depression and mania. *Lancet* **2**, 108.

Rawls, W. E. (1973). Herpes simplex virus. *In* "The Herpes Viruses" (Ed. A. S. Kaplan). Academic Press, New York and London.

Regnier, E. (1968). The administration of large doses of ascorbic acid in the prevention and treatment of the common cold, Part I. *Review of Allergy* **22**, 835-846.

Regnier, E. (1968). The administration of large doses of ascorbic acid in the prevention and treatment of the common cold, Part II. *Review of Allergy* **22**, 948-975.

Rhead, W. J. and Schrauzer, G. N. (1971). Risks of long-term ascorbic acid overdosage. *Nutrition Reviews* **29**, 262-263.

Ritzel, Von G. (1961). Kritische Beurteilung des Vitamins C als Prophylacticum und Therapeuticum der Erkältungskrankheiten. *Helv. Med. Acta* **28**, 63.

Robinson, G. A., Butcher, R. W. and Sutherland, E. W. (1971). "Cyclic AMP", Academic Press, New York and London.

Roe, J. H. (1954-5). "Methods of Biochemical Analysis", I, pp. 115-139. (Ed. D. Glick). Wiley, New York.

Roe, J. H. (1961). Appraisal of methods for the determination of L-ascorbic acid. *Annals. N.Y. Acad. Sci.* **92**, 277.

Roe, J. H. and Kuether, C. A. (1943). The determination of ascorbic acid in whole blood and urine through the 2,4-Dinitrophenylhydrazine derivative of dehydroascorbic acid. *J. Biol Chem.* **147**, 399-407.

Roe, J. H. and Itscoitz, S. B. (1963). Studies on binding of ascorbic acid in animal tissues. *Proc. Soc. Exptl. Biol. and Med.* **113**, 648-650.

Rosenthal, G. (1971). Interaction of ascorbic acid and warfarin. *J. Amer. Med. Assoc.* **215**, 1671.

Roston, S. (1962). Ascorbic acid, oxygen and the disappearance of adreno-chrome and noradrenochrome. *Nature* **194**, 1079-1080.

Roston, S. (1965). Studies of the epinephrine-glutathione reaction in aqueous solution and human blood. *Arch. Biochem. Biophys.* **109**, 41-48.

Roy, R. N. and Guha, B. C. (1958). Species difference in regard to the biosynthesis of ascorbic acid. *Nature (Lond.)* **182**, 319-320.

Rudolff, S. L., Becker, R. R. and King, C. G. (1956). Synthesis and metabolism of L-ascorbic acid-2,3,4,5,6-C^{14}. *Fed. Proceed.* **15**, 343.

Ruskin, A. and Ruskin, B. (1952). Effect of mercurial diuretics upon the respiration of the rat heart and kidney. *Texas Reports on Biology and Medicine* **10**, 429-438.

Russell, G. A., Strom, E. T., Talaty, E. R., Chang, K. Y., Stephens, R. D. and Young, M. C. (1966). Application of electron spin resonance spectroscopy problems of structure and conformation. Aliphatic semidiones. *Rec. Chem. Progress* **27**, 3-35.

Ryan, W. L. and Coronel. D. M. (1969). Adenosine 3',5'-monophophosphate as an inhibitor of ovulation and reproduction. *Amer. J. Obstetrics and Gynecol.* **105**, 121-123.

Ryan, W. L. and Heidrick, M. L. (1968). Inhibition of cell growth in vitro by adenosine 3',5'-monophosphate. *Science* **162**, 1484-1485.

S

Sabin, A. B. (1939). Vitamin C in relation to experimental poliomyelitis. *J. Exptl. Med.* **69**, 507-515.

Sahagian, B. M., Harding-Barlow, I. and Mitchell Perry, H. (1967). Transmural movements of zinc, manganese, cadmium and mercury by rat intestine. *J. Nutrition* **93**, 291–300.

Sasmal, N., Mukherjee, D., Kar, N. C. and Chatterjee, G. C. (1968). Effect of manganese and cobalt on ascorbic acid metabolism in rats. *Ind. J. Biochem.* **5**, 123–125.

Schaus, R. (1957). The ascorbic acid content of human pituitary, cerebral cortex, heart and skeletal muscle and its relation to age. *Amer. J. Clin. Nutrition* **5**, 39–31.

Schayer, R. W. (1962). Evidence that induced histamine is an intrinsic regulator of the microcirculatory system. *Am. J. Physiol.* **202**, 66–72.

Schjeide, O. A. and De Vellis, J. (1970). "Cell Differentiation" Van Nostrand Reinhold Co.

Schirmacher, H. and Schneider, J. (1955). Grenzen und Möglichkeiten der Vitamin-A- und C-Übervitaminierung bei inoperablen und strahlenresistenten Karzinomen. *Zeitschrift für Geburtshilfe und Gynaekologie* (*Stuttgart*). **144**, 172–182.

Schneider, E. (1955). Abwehrvorgänge gegen Tumore im Spiegel einer Hautreaktion. *Wiener Medizinische Wochenschrift* **20/21**, 430–432.

Schneider, E. (1954). Vitamin C und A beim Karzinom. *Deutsche med. Wochenschrift* **79**, 15, 584–587.

Schneider, E. (1956). Hypervitamin therapy of cancer. *Medizinische*, 183–187.

Schneider, W. and Staudinger, Hj. (1965). Reduced nicotinamide-adenine dinucleotide dependent reduction of semidehydroascorbic acid. *Biochim. Biophys. Acta* **96**, 157–159.

Schubert, J. and Lindenbaum, A. (1952). Stability of alkaline earth-organic acid complexes measured by ion exchange. *J. Amer. Chem. Soc.* **74**, 3529–3532.

Schultz, C., Hardman, J. G. and Sutherland, E. W. (1973). *In* "Asthma. Physiology, Pharmacology and Treatment", Chapter 9. "Cyclic Nucleotides and Smooth Muscle Function", pp. 123–138. Academic Press, London and New York.

Schwab, M. and Khuns, K. (1959). "Die Störungen des Wasser- und Elektrolytstoffwechsels", Springer-Verlag, Berlin.

Schwartz, A. R., Togo, Y., Hornick, R. B., Tominaga, S. and Gleckman, R. A. (1973). Evaluation of the efficacy of ascorbic acid in prophylaxis of induced rhinovirus 44 infection in man. *J. Infectious Diseases* **128**, 500–505.

Scott, R. E. (1970). Effect of prostaglandines, epinephrine and NaF on human leucocyte, platelet and liver adenyl cyclase. *Blood* **35**, 514–516.

Secher, K. (1942). The bearing of the ascorbic acid content of the blood on the course of the blood sugar curve. *Acta Medica Scandinavia* **60**, II–III, 255–265.

Seelert, K. and Schenk, G. (1966). Polarographische Untersuchungen der Ascorbinsäure-Oxydation durch Chinone. *Archiv. für Pharmazie* (*Weinheim*) **299**, 757–762.

Senft, G., Schultz, G., Munske, K. and Hoffman, M. (1968). Influence of insulin on cyclic 3',5'-AMP phosphodiesterase activity in liver, skeletal muscle, adipose tissue, and kidney. *Diabetologia* **4**, 322–329.

Shaffer, C. F. (1944). The diuretic effect of ascorbic acid. *J. Amer. Med. Assoc.* **124**, 700–701.

Shaffer, C. F. (1970). Ascorbic acid and atherosclerosis. *Am. J. Clin. Nutrition* **23**, 27–30.

Shapiro, S. S. and Bishop, M. (1975). Effect of ascorbic acid on hyaluronidase inhibitor. *Nature* **253**, 479–480.

Sharma, S. K., Johnstone, R. M. and Quastel, J. H. (1963). Active transport of ascorbic acid in adrenal cortex and brain cortex *in vitro* and the effects of ACTH and steroids. *Canadian J. of Biochem. and Physiol.* **41**, 597–604.

Sherry, S. and Ralli, E. P. (1948). Further studies of the effects of insulin on the metabolism of vitamin C. *J. Clin. Invest.* **27**, 217–225.

Shimazono, N. and Mano, Y. (1961). Enzymatic studies on the metabolism of uronic and aldonic acids related to L-ascorbic acid in animal tissues. *Ann. N.Y. Acad. Sci.* **92**, 91–104.

Shimizu, H., Daly, J. W. and Creveling, C. R. (1969). A radioisotopic method for measuring the formation of adenosine 3',5'-cyclic monophosphate in incubated slices of brain. *J. Neurochem.* **16**, 1609–1619.

Sigell, L. T. and Flessa, H. C. (1940). Drug interactions with anticoagulants. *J. Amer. Med. Assoc.* **214**, 2035–2039.

Spero, L. and Anderson, T. W. (1973). Ascorbic acid and common colds. *Brit. Med. J.* **4**, 354.

Smith, H. W. (1951). "The Kidney; Structure and Function in Health and Disease". Oxford University Press, New York.

Sokoloff, B., Hori, M., Saelhof, C. C., Wrzokek, T. and Imai, T. (1966). Ageing, atherosclerosis and ascorbic acid metabolism. *J. Am. Gereat. Soc.* **14**, No. 12, 1239–1260.

Sokoloff, B., Hori, M., Saelohf, C., McConnell, B. and Imai, T. (1967). Effect of ascorbic acid on certain blood fat metabolism factors in animals and men. *J. of Nutrition* **91**, 107–118.

Spellberg, M. A. and Meeton, R. W. (1939). Ascorbic acid in relation to saturation and utilization with some diabetic implications. *Arch. Int. Med.* **63**, 1095–1116.

Spero, L. (1974). Quoted by Lewin, S. (1974). in *Chemistry in Britain* **10**, 25–27.

Spittle, C. R. (1971). Atherosclerosis and vitamin C. *Lancet* 1280–1281.

Spittle, C. R. (1972). Atherosclerosis and vitamin C. *Lancet* **1**, 1335.

Srivastava, G. C. and Sirohi, G. S. (1969). Effect of ascorbic acid on transamination of glutamic acid and alanine. *Ind. J. Exptl. Biol.* **7**, 129–130.

Stepp, N. and Schroder, H. (1936). Über die Beziehungen des Vitamin C zum Stoffwechsel des Carcinomgewebes. *Ztschr, f.d. ges. exper. Med.* **98**, 611–622.

Stern, H. and Timonen, S. (1954). The position of the cell nucleus in pathways of hydrogen transfer: cytochrome c, flavoproteins, glutathione and ascorbic acid. *J. Gen. Physiol.* **48**, 41–52.

Stone, I. (1966). Hypoascorbemia. The genetic disease causing the human requirement for exogenous ascorbic acid. *Perspectives Mo. Biol.* **10**, 133-134.

Stone, I. (1972). The healing factor. *In* "Vitamin C against Disease". Crosset and Dunlap, New York.

Storey, I. D. E. and Dutton, G. J. (1955). Uridine compounds in glucuronic acid metabolism. *Biochem. J.* **59**, 279-288.

Strominger, J. L., Kalckar, H. M., Axelrod, J. and Maxwell, E. S. (1954). Enzymatic oxidation of uridine diphosphate glucose to uridine diphosphate glucuronic acid. *J. Amer. Chem. Soc.* **76**, 6411-6412.

Subramanian, N., Nandi, B. K., Majumder, A. K. and Chatterjee, I. B. (1973). Role of L-ascorbic acid on detoxification of histamine. *Biochemical Pharmacology* **22**, 1671-1673.

Sumerwell, W. N. and Sealocki, R. R. (1952). The determination of bound ascorbic acid in liver tissue. *J. Biol. Chem.* **196**, 753-759.

Sure, B. (1932). Avitaminosis. XI. The specific effect of vitamin B on growth as evidenced by the use of vitamin B concentrate. *J. Biol. Chem.* **97**, 133-139.

Sussman, K. E. and Vaughan, G. D. (1967). Insulin release after ACTH, glucagon and adenosine-3',5'-phosphate (cyclic AMP) in the perfused isolated rat pancreas. *Diabetes* **16**, 449-452.

Sutherland, E. W. (1956). Proc. 3rd Int. Congr. Biochem. pp. 318-327. Academic Press, New York.

Svirbely, J. L. (1936). The effect of diets and various substances on the vitamin C content of some organs of the rat. *Amer. J. Physiology* **116**, 446-455.

Sylvest, O. (1942). The effect of ascorbic acid on the carbohydrate metabolism. *Acta Medica Scand.* **60**, II-III, 183-189.

Szenes, T. (1942). Die Wirkung der Ascorbinsäure bei der Röntgenbestrahlung von Geschwülsten und geschwulstartigen Wucherungen. *Strahlen Therapie* **71**, 463-471.

Szent-Györgyi, A. (1968). Bioelectronics. Intermolecular electron transfer may play a major role in biological regulation, defense and cancer. *Science* **161**, 988-990.

T

Tagi-Zade, S. B. (1961). Vitamin C exchange in cancerous patients during radium therapy. *Meditsinskaia Radiologia* **6**, 10-16 (Russian).

Takiguchi, H., Furuyama, S. and Shimazono, N. (1966). Urinary oxalic acid excretion by man following ingestion of large amounts of ascorbic acid. *J. of Vitaminology* **12**, 307-312.

Tappel, A. L. (1965). Free radical lipid peroxidation damage and its inhibition by vitamin E and selenium. *Fed. Proceed.* **24**, 73-78.

Tappel, A. L. (1968). Will antioxidant nutrients slow ageing processes? *Geriatrics* **23**, Part 10, 97-105.

Tarro, G. and Sabin, A. B. (1973). Nonvirion antigens produced by Herpes simplex viruses 1 and 2. *Proc. Nat. Acad. Sci. U.S.A.* **70**, 1032-1036.

Thornton, P. A. (1968). Bone salt mobilization effected by ascorbic acid. *Proc. Soc. for Experimental Biology and Medicine* **127**, 1096-1099.

Thornton, P. A. (1970). Influence of exogenous ascorbic acid on calcium and phosphorus metabolism of the chick. *J. Nutrition* **100**, 1479–1486.

Tiapina, L. A. (1961). L'effet de l'acide ascorbique sur les lipides sanguins dans l'hypertension essentielle et l'atherosclerose. *Cor et Vasa* **3**(2):98–106.

Tisdale, M. J. (1975). Inhibition of cyclic adenosine 3′,5′-monophosphate phosphodiesterase from Walker carcinoma by ascorbic and dehydroascorbic acids. *Biochem. Biophys. Res. Commun.* **61**, 877–881.

Todhunter, E. N., Robbins, R. C. and McIntosh, J. A. (1942). The rate of increase of blood plasma ascorbic acid after ingestion of ascorbic acid (Vitamin C). *J. Nutrition* **23**, 309–319.

Tolbert, B. M., Chen, A. W., Bell, E. M. and Baker, E. M. (1967). Metabolism of L-ascorbic-4-³H acid in man. *Am. J. of Clin. Nutrition* **20**, 250–252.

Tolbert, B. M., Downing, M., Carlson, R. W., Knight, M. K. and Baker, E. M. (1975). Chemistry and metabolism of ascorbic acid and ascorbic sulphate. *Ann. N.Y. Acad. Sci.* (Vitamin C Conference, October 1974).

Touster, O., Reynolds, V. H. and Hutcheson, R. M. (1956). The reduction of L-xylulose to xylitol by guinea pig liver mitochondria. *J. Biol. Chem.* **221**, 697–709.

Touster, O. and Hollmann, S. (1961). Nutritional and enzymatic studies on the mechanism of stimulation of ascorbic acid synthesis by drugs and carcinogenic hydrocarbons. *Ann. N.Y. Acad. Sci.* **92**, 318–323.

Turtle, J. R. and Kipnis, D. M. (1967). An adrenergic receptor mechanism for the control of cyclic 3′,5′-adenosine monophosphate synthesis in tissues. *Biochem. Biophys. Res. Commun.* **28**, 797–802.

U

Udenfriend, S., Clark, C. T., Axelrod, J. and Brodie, B. B. (1954). Ascorbic acid in aromatic hydroxylation. I. A model system for aromatic hydroxylation. *J. Biol. Chem.* **208**, 731–739.

V

Van Wyk, C. P. and Kotze, J. P. (1975). Effect of ascorbic acid on plasma adenosine 3′,5′-cyclic monophosphate level in the baboon, Papio Ursinus. *South African J. of Science* **71**, 28–29.

Verlangieri, A. J. and Mumma, R. O. (1973). *In vivo* sulfation of cholesterol by ascorbic acid 2-sulfate. *Atherosclerosis* **17**, 37–48.

Versteeg, J. (1969). Effect of ascorbic acid on virus replication, and production and activity of interferon in vitro. Proc. Koninkl. *Nederl. Akad. Wetensch.* (*Biol. Med.*) **72**, 207–212.

Vogt, A. (1940). Zur Vitamin C-Behandlung der chronischen Leukämien. *Deutsche Medizinische Wochenschrift* **66**, 369–372.

W

Waelsch, H. and Rackow, H. (1942). Natural and synthetic inhibitors of choline esterase. *Science* **96**, 386.

Waldo, A. L. and Zipf, R. E. (1955). Ascorbic acid level in leukemic patients. *Cancer* **8**, 187-190.

Walker, G. H., Bynoe, M. L. and Tyrrell, D. A. J. (1967). Trial of ascorbic acid in prevention of colds. *Brit. Med. J.* **1**, 603-606.

Walters, C. L. (1974). 6. Vitamin C and nitrosamine formation. *In* "Vitamin C. Recent Aspects of its Physiological and Technological Importance" (Ed. G. G. Birch and K. Parker.)

Walters, C. L. and Taylor, A. McM. (1964). Nitrite metabolism by muscle *in vitro. Biochim. Biophys. Acta* **86**, 448-458.

Warren, F. L. (1943). Aerobic oxidation of aromatic hydrocarbons in presence of ascorbic acid. *Biochem. J.* **37**, 338-341.

Watson, A. F. (1943). Chemical reducing capacity and vitamin C content of transplantable tumors of rat and guinea pig. *Brit. J. Exp. Pathol.* **17**, 124-134.

Weis, W. (1974/5). "Ascorbic Acid and Electron Transport". Abstracts of 2nd Vitamin C Conference (1974). *Ann. N.Y. Acad. Sci.*

Weissberger, A. and Lu Valle, J. E. (1944). The autoxidation of ascorbic acid in the presence of copper. *J. Amer. Chem. Soc.* **66**, 701-705.

Williams, R. J. (1963). The basis for the genetotrophic concept. *In* "Biochemical Individuality". John Wiley and Sons, New York.

Williams, R. J. and Deason, G. (1967). Individuality in vitamin C needs. *Proc. Natnl. Acad. Sci., U.S.A.* **57**, 1638-1641.

Willis, G. C. (1957). The reversibility of atherosclerosis. *Canad. M. A. J.* **77**, 106-109.

Willis, G. C. and Fishman, S. (1955). Ascorbic acid content of human arterial tissue. *Canad. M. A. J.* **72**, 500-503.

Wise, E. M., Alexander, S. P. and Powers, M. (1973). Adenosine $3':5'$-cyclic monophosphate as a regulator of bacterial transformation. *Proc. Nat. Acad. Sci. U.S.A.* **70**, 471-474.

Wilson, C. W. M. and Loh, H. S. (1969). Ascorbic acid and upper respiratory inflammation. *Acta Allergologica* **XXIV**, 367-380.

Wilson, C. W. M. and Loh, H. S. (1973). Common cold and vitamin C. *Lancet* **638-641**.

Wilson, C. W. M. and Loh, H. S. (1973). Vitamin C and fertility. *Lancet* **859-860**.

Wilson, W. M. W. (1973). Ascorbic acid and the common cold. *Brit. Med. J.* **166-167**.

Woodward, G. E. (1935). Glutathione and ascorbic acid in tissues of normal and tumor-bearing albino rats. *Biochem. J.* **29**, 2405-2412.

Woolum, J. C., Tiezzi, E. and Commoner, B. (1968). Electron spin resonance of iron-nitric oxide complexes with amino acids, peptides and proteins. *Biochim. Biophys. Acta* **160**, 311-320.

Y

Yamazaki, I., Mason, H. S. and Piette, L. (1959). Identification of intermediate substrate free-radicals formed during peroxidatic oxidations, by electron paramagnetic resonance spectroscopy. *Biochem. Biophys. Res. Commun.* **1**, No. 6, 336–337.

Yamazaki, I., Mason, H. S. and Piette, L. (1960). Identification, by electron paramagnetic resonance spectroscopy, of free radicals generated from substrates by peroxidase. *J. Biol. Chem.* **235**, 2444–2449.

Yamazaki, I. and Piette, L. H. (1961). Mechanism of free radical formation and disappearance during the ascorbic acid oxidase and peroxidase reactions. *Biochim. Biophys. Acta* **50**, 62–69.

Yamazaki, I. (1962). The reduction of cytochrome c by enzyme-generated ascorbic free radical. *J. Biol. Chem.* **237**, 224–229.

Yavorsky, M., Almaden, P. and King, C. G. (1934). The Vitamin C content of human tissues. *J. Biol. Chem.* **106**, 525–529.

Yew, M. L. (1973). Recommended daily allowances for vitamin C. *Proc. Nat. Acad. Sci.* **70**, 4, 969–972.

Yew, M. L. (1975). "Biological Variation in Ascorbic Acid Needs." Second International Conference on Vitamin C held in New York 9–12 Oct. 1974. *Ann. N.Y. Acad. Sci.*

Z

Zuck, D. A. and Conine, J. W. (1963). Stabilisation of vitamin B_{12} I. Complex cyanides. *Jnl. Pharmaceutical Sciences* **52**, 59–63.

Zureick, M. (1950). Traitement du zona et de l'herpes par la vitamine C intraveineuse. *Journal des Praticiens* **64**, 586.

Zuskin, E., Lewis, A. J. and Bouhuys, A. (1973). Inhibition of histamine-induced airway constriction by ascorbic acid. *J. Allergy Clin. Immunol.* **51**, 218–226.

Bibliography

It was not practical to include various relevant references in the treatment undertaken in the main part of the book; these are included in the following Bibliography. Additionally, information on various aspects of ascorbic acid structure, synthesis and involvement can be obtained from the following Bibliography giving lists of major conferences and review articles.

I. Conferences

(a) "First Conference on Vitamin C" held in New York (1961), Proceedings published in *Ann. N.Y. Acad. Sci.* **94**.

(b) 11th Symposium held by the Deuttschen Gesellschaft fur Ernährung in Mainz, 2nd to 3rd April, 1964, entitled "Ascorbinsäure". Published in "Wissenschaflitche Veroffentlichungen der Deutschen Gessellschaft für Ernährung, Vol. 14". Dr. Dietrich Steinkipff Verlag, Darmstadt, 1965.

(c) "Vitamin C and the Common Cold" Symposium, held as the Seventh Industrial Affilates Symposium at Stanford University, August 6–7, 1973. A report of the Conference was given by S. Lewin in *Chemistry in Britain* (1974), **10**, 25–27.

(d) "First International Symposium on Vitamin C". An industry–university co-operation Symposium organized under the auspices of the National College of Food Technology, University of Reading, on 2nd and 3rd April, 1974. The Proceedings were published in "Vitamin C. Recent Aspects of its Physiological and Technological Importance". Eds. G. C. Birch and K. J. Parker (1974). Applied Science Publishers, London.

(e) "Second Conference on Vitamin C", organized by the New York Academy of Sciences and held in New York on 9–12 October, 1974. *Ann. N.Y. Acad. Sci.* (1975).

II. Major reviews and articles on various aspects of Vitamin C

(a) Rosenberg, H. (1942). *In* "Chemistry and Physiology of the Vitamins", 289–338. Interscience, New York.

(b) Lloyd, B. B. and Sinclair, H. M. (1953). *In* "Biochemistry and Physiology of Nutrition, I", Chapter 11. Vitamin C. 369–471. Academic Press, New York and London.

(c) Gould, B. S. (1963). Collagen formation and fibrogenesis with special reference to the role of ascorbic acid. *Internat. Rev. Cytol.* **15**, 301–361.

(d) Ross, R. and Benditt, E. P. (1964). Wound healing and collagen formation. IV. Distortion of ribosomal patterns of fibroblasts in scurvy. *J. Cell Biology* **22**, 365–389.

(e) Woodruff, C. W. (1964). Ascorbic acid, Chapter 4. "Nutrition", 265–298.

(f) Shimizu, Y., McCann, D. S. and Keech, M. K. (1965). The effect of ascorbic acid on human dermal fibroblasts in monolayer tissue culture. *J. Lab. Clinical Med.* 286–306.

(g) Udenfriend, S. (1966). Formation of hydroxyproline in collagen. *Science* **152**, 1335–1340.

(h) Burns, J. J. Ascorbic acid, Chapter 7. "Metabolic Pathways", Vol. I, 3rd Edn. (Ed. D. H. Greenberg). Academic Press, London and New York.

(i) Sebrell, W. H. and Harris, R. S. (1967). Chapter 2, entitled "Ascorbic Acid", 306–385, contains several contributions by Harris, R. S., Hay, G. W., Lewis, B. A., Smith, F., Oliver, M., Mapson, L. W., Chatterjee, G. C. and Vilter, R. W.

(j) Barnes, M. J. and Kodicek, E. (1972). Biological hydroxylations and ascorbic acid with special reference to collagen metabolism. *Vitamins and Hormones* **30**, 1–43.

(k) Tauber, H. (1938). The interaction of ascorbic acid (Vitamin C) with enzymes. *Ergebn. Enzymforschung* **7**, 301–315.

(l) Anon. (1973). Ascorbate stimulation of tyrosine hydroxylase formation. *Nutrition Reviews* **31**, 93.

(m) Anon. (1973b). Activation of prolyl hydroxylase by ascorbic acid. *Nutrition Reviews* **31**, 255–256.

(n) Silbert, N. E. (1951). Vitamin C. A critical review of the use of vitamin C in allergic disorders and a preliminary report comparing it therapeutically with antihistamines, antiasthmatics and sedatives. *Med. Times* **79**, 370–376.

(o) Goldsmith, G. A., Ogaard, A. T. and Gowe, D. F. (1941). Vitamin C (ascorbic acid). Nutrition in bronchial asthma. *Arch. Intern. Med.* **67**, 597–608.

(p) Mazur, A., Baez, S. and Shorr, E. (1955). The mechanism of iron release from ferritin as related to its biological properties. *J. Biol. Chem.* **213**, 147–160.

(q) Mazur, A., Green, S. and Carleton, A. (1960). Mechanism of plasma iron incorporation into hepatic ferritin. *J. Biol. Chem.* **235**, 595–603.

(r) Mazur, A. (1961). Role of ascorbic acid in the incorporation of plasma iron into ferritin. *Ann. N.Y. Acad. Sci.* **92**, 223–229.

III. Assay of vitamin C and its products

(1) *General Chemical Methods*

(a) Roe, J. H. (1954–5). Chemical determination of ascorbic, dehydroascorbic and digluconic acids. *In* "Methods of Biochemical Analysis". Vol. I, pp. 115–138 (Ed. D. Glick). Wiley, New York.

(b) Rosenberg, H. R. (1945). *In* "Chemistry and Physiology of the Vitamins", pp. 316–322. Interscience, New York and London.

(c) Cooke, J. R. (1974). The chemical estimation of vitamin C. *In* "Vitamin C. Recent Advances of its Physiological and Technical Importance", pp. 31–39. (Eds. G. C. Birch and K. Parker). Applied Science Publishers, London.

(d) Mammie Oliver, Estimation of ascorbic acid. A review. *In* "The Vitamins, Vol. I", 2nd Edn. pp. 338–359.

(2) *Methods utilizing ascorbic oxidase*

(a) Marchesini, A., Polesselo, A. and Zoja, G. (1970). Dosaggio enzimatico dell'acido ascorbico nei vegetali freschi e conservati. *Agrochimia* **14**, 453–461.

(b) Marchesini, A. and Manitto, P. (1972). Un nuovo metodo enzimatico per dosare l'acido ascorbico, deidroascorbico ed i riduttoni nei vegetali freschi e conservati. *Agrochimia* 16, 351–361.

(3) *Fluorimetric methods based on the reaction between Dehydroascorbic and Ortho-phenylenediamine*
(a) Deutsch, M. J. and Weeks, C. E. (1965). Microfluorometric assay for Vitamin C. *J. Assoc. Off. Agric. Chem.* 48, (6), 1248–1256.
(b) "Official Methods of Analysis of the Association of Official Analytical Chemists", 11th edn. (1970). *Microfluorimetric Methods.* 778, 779, AOAC, Washington, D.C.
(c) Davidek, J., Velisek, J. and Nezbedova, M. (1971). Determination of dehydroascorbic acid in meat and meat products. *Sb. Vys. Sk. Chem.- Technol. Praze Potraviny* E30, 17–23.

(4) *Column, paper and thin layer chromatographic separations from other substances*
(a) Crossland, I. (1960). Chromatographic determination of ascorbic acid. *Acta Chem. Scand.* 14(4), 805–813.
(b) Hegenauer, J. and Saltman, P. (1972). Resolution of ascorbic dehydro-ascorbic and digketogulonic acids by anion-exchange column chromatography. *J. Chromatog.* 74(1), 133–137.

(5) *Gas chromatography of silylated ascorbic acid and dehydroascorbic acid*
(a) Sweeley, C. G., Bentley, R., Makita, M. and Wells, W. (1963). Gas-liquid chromatography of trimethylsilyl derivatives of sugars and related substances. *J. Amer. Chem. Soc.* 85, 2497–2507.
(b) Pfeilsticker, K. (1968). Gas chromatographie der L-ascorbinsäure und dehydroascorbinsäure. *Fresnius' Z. anal. Chem.* 237(2), 97–103.
(c) Allison, J. H. and Stewart, M. A. (1971). Quantitative analysis of ascorbic acid in tissues by gas-liquid chromatography. *Analyt. Biochem.* 43, 401–409.

(6) *Radioactive tracer assay*
(a) Baker, E. M., Levandoski, V. G. and Sauberlich, H. E. (1963). Respiratory catabolism in man of the degradative intermediates of L-ascorbic-1-C^{14} acid. *Proc. Soc. Exptl. Biol. Med.* 113, 379–383.
(b) Saari, J. C., Baker, E. M. and Sauberlich, H. E. (1967). Thin layer chromatographic separation of the oxidative degradation products of ascorbic acid. *Analyt. Biochem.* 18, 173–177.

(7) *Books*
(a) "Ascorbimetric Titrations", L. Erdey and G. Svehla, Akademiai Kiado, Budapest, 1973.

Index

W

Warfarin, 171
Water,
    ascorbate, and, 16
    bulk water, 15, 26, 48, 60
    free radicals, 35, 36

X

Xylulose fork, 108, 113

Z

Zwitterion, 34